THE
INTERIOR
SILENCE

THE

INTERIOR

SILENCE

My Encounters with Calm, Joy, and Compassion
at 10 Monasteries Around the World

SARAH SANDS

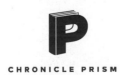

CHRONICLE PRISM

First published in the United States of America in 2021
by Chronicle Books LLC.
Originally published in the United Kingdom in 2021
by Short Books, an imprint of Octopus Publishing Group Ltd.

Library of Congress Cataloging-in-Publication Data available.

ISBN 978-1-7972-1045-2

Manufactured in the United States of America.

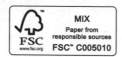

Design by Brooke Johnson.
Illustrations by Evie Dunne.
Typesetting by Maureen Forys, Happenstance Type-O-Rama.
Typeset in Adobe Caslon Pro and Sackers.

10 9 8 7 6 5 4 3 2 1

Chronicle books and gifts are available at special quantity
discounts to corporations, professional associations, literacy
programs, and other organizations. For details and discount
information, please contact our premiums department at
corporatesales@chroniclebooks.com or at 1-800-759-0190.

CHRONICLE PRISM

Chronicle Prism is an imprint of Chronicle Books LLC,
680 Second Street, San Francisco, California 94107

www.chronicleprism.com

To Tilly, for teaching me by example

CONTENTS

PREFACE

O n a winter's day, in which the sky hangs like a flat sheet over Norfolk, I look out at the remains of a thirteenth-century monastery wall in the field at the edge of my garden. Yew trees and ivy form a dark green curtain around the chalk-gray stone. There are two stone windows, in the shapes of a four- and six-leaf clover, and some smaller holes beneath. Sometimes jackdaws dart out of these holes, and earlier in the year I heard harsh squeals. I crept toward the sound and found massively dilated eyes in flat, fetal faces staring out at me. In time, the baby barn owls fledged and flew.

Behind the wall are hazel and walnut trees; in January, sun-yellow aconites; February, a mass of snowdrops; in March, primroses; April, bluebells; then foxgloves, ferns, and a crescendo of summer fecundity—poppies, nettles, cow parsley. I use a hacked branch of hazel to slash through a path. Its bark has been gnawed by the deer that leap over the field fence.

The wall is all that remains of Marham Abbey—a Cistercian nunnery destroyed by Henry VIII's marital ambitions and schism with Rome. It went in the first wave, because it had no bargaining power. It was poor, and it housed women.

A wall and a cascade of discarded stones. Some of these were used in Victorian times to build my hodgepodge house. I have kept various larger pieces of masonry as doorstops, and on the mantelpiece are a couple of glazed tiles, one pattern worn to yellow on a russet background. The shape could be many things but I trace it as an oak tree. The other is a much more detailed edging of medieval crosses and symbols.

When a friend and Norfolk neighbor, who is also an expert in historic buildings, came to see the house, he declared some of the brickwork in the chimney of historical interest. It was Tudor, retained by the Victorian builders. There was "nothing else of note." I remember the term whenever I become too enthusiastic about the place. The wall is a scheduled monument, which means that you cannot build on it, but the house is not even listed by the conservation authorities. Henry VIII certainly found nothing of note here. The total loot was worth forty-six pounds (sixty-three dollars).

Yet the wall exists as a center of gravity in my life, and the lessons of monastic life are contained within it. The Cistercian order followed the teachings of the French abbot Bernard of Clairvaux, who said: "You will find in woods something you will never find in books—stones and trees will teach you a lesson you never heard in the schools."

The great English Cistercian monastery is Rievaulx Abbey in North Yorkshire.

I read about it because my wall is a poor relation, and I want to know about the distant and grandest Cistercian community. It is about a five-hour drive from my home, and one day I set off with an inexplicable sense of purpose.

My route takes me past Lincoln Cathedral, rising like a thunderous organ from the flat landscape. I say to myself: "I lift up mine eyes."

I drive on, listening to one of Bach's *Brandenburg Concertos* on the radio, along a monotonous road until I pass Wakefield, Leeds, Ripon, Helmsley. Then the roads become narrow and I miss several times the unmarked, unmade route, which is almost like a farm drive, past miles of skeleton trees, descending into a remote valley of the river Rye in the North Yorkshire moors. The hidden nature of Rievaulx makes its revelation all the more heart-stopping.

Alone, I wander through the vistas of columns and framed views of stirring Yorkshire countryside. I imagine the first monks who sheltered here under the rocks of the valley and among the elm trees.

The remoteness of monasteries—best viewed from the heavens—is in their essence; it is a rejection of the material world, its rhythms and its values. The monks lived by sunrise and sunset and spent their time between in learning, meditation, and manual labor. This inner concentration buoyed them in an extraordinary weightlessness. Saint Aelred, abbot of Rievaulx monastery, said: "Everywhere peace, everywhere serenity, and a marvelous freedom from the tumult of the world."

When I returned from Rievaulx, I was changed. I saw my wall in a different light—easy to do, for the relationship between solid stone and the canvas of the skies is an everlasting painting. My sense of kinship with it deepened and my curiosity tingled. I saw that it was part of a network of monasteries across the country; ruined, silent, consigned to history—they all had stories to tell. There was wisdom in these institutions and there was medicine, for the body and for the mind. After all, out of the monasteries came both universities and hospitals, our most humane and valued institutions.

The principle of caring for the ill was cited by Shenoute, the third-century Egyptian monk: "It is he [God] who will judge anyone who scorns those who are sick among us and among you." Furthermore, the monks showed an early understanding of what we now call mental health. Illness is not always visible. Many things of meaning cannot be seen, such as love. Another quote from the desert fathers—those who first founded monasteries in the scorched emptiness of Egypt—is this: "Nor let us speak insults to one another, such as 'You are not sick,' lest God be angry with us because of our ignorance. For who knows what is inside man other than the Lord."

If monks fell ill, they would be cared for, while they were expected to exhibit stoicism in the face of sickness. Both knowledge of surgery and stoicism put monks at an advantage. Here is an account of a monk named Abba Aaronin from sixth-century Constantinople:

> *Once Aaron fell under a serious disease of gangrene in his loins; and he bore this affliction with great discretion, until his penis was eaten up and mutilated and had vanished down to its root, and his disease began to enter his inner organs. . . . But he, for his part, until his wound had worsened severely, held fast—constant*

in prayer and filling his mouth with praise and thanksgiving to God. Finally, when he could no longer pass water he was forced and so persuaded to reveal and make known his disease. Then the whole of his penis was found eaten away and consumed so that the physicians contrived to make a tube of lead and placed it for the passing of his water, while also applying bandages and drugs to him. And so the ulcer was healed. Furthermore, Aaron lived eighteen years after the crisis of this test, praising God, and having that lead tube in place for the necessity of passing water.

It has taken a global pandemic today to remind us that affliction is part of life, although the symptoms are less grisly.

The monastic way of living intrigued me—it had become a secret corner of my life. My work is in London, but Norfolk is my place of sanctuary. The wall represents something antithetical to my London life. It is the still, small voice that provides a contrast to the needy, WhatsApping, power-conscious world of politics and media.

The job that I had until September 2020 was to edit the BBC's flagship news and current affairs show, the *Today* program, during the most politically and socially fractious of periods. People were angry about whether or not Britain should leave the European Union, and the *Today* program was a lightning rod. Furthermore, I was responsible for the running order of the program, which was a work in progress over twenty-four hours. My phone beeped incessantly. There were months when it buzzed hysterically between 3:00 A.M. and 5:00 A.M., until I realized that, apart from all the journalistic messages, I had somehow become the switchboard for all the taxis ordered by the BBC news department.

Skimming six hours' sleep a night and ever part of a jittery and constant news conversation, I was finding it hard to switch off. One night during which I simply could not sleep, I picked up a book.

It was a slim volume, called *A Time to Keep Silence*, by the great adventurer Patrick Leigh Fermor. I had read all his books except for this one, considering it an aberration. Who cared about silence? Life was best lived at the center of events, not at the margins.

I was sorry to have been born into a different age than Leigh Fermor, and indeed I had an unseemly crush on him, considering that he was dead.

He was described by one of his teachers as a "dangerous mixture of sophistication and recklessness." His life was of celebrated daring and pleasure.

Yet, he was drawn to monasteries. *A Time to Keep Silence*, published in 1957, is an account of his sojourns at three of them: the Abbey of Saint Wandrille, Solesmes Abbey, and La Grande Trappe. In the book, Leigh Fermor confessed to depression and anxiety; he yearned for peace and stillness. As the monks would say, who knows what is inside man other than the Lord?

I read his prose, puzzled. The man I understood to be conqueringly urbane wrote:

> *In spite of private limitations I was profoundly affected by the places I have described. . . . The kindness of the monks has something to do with this. But more important was the discovery of a capacity for solitude and (on however humble a level compared to that of most people who resort to monasteries) for the recollectedness and clarity of spirit that accompany the silent monastic life.*

He also experienced a higher plane of sleeping:

After initial spells of insomnia, nightmare and falling asleep by day, I found that my capacity for sleep became more remarkable and my sleep was so profound that I might have been under the influence of some hypnotic drug. . . . Then began an extraordinary transformation: night shrank to five hours of light, dreamless and perfect sleep, followed by awakenings full of energy and limpid freshness.

Can you imagine that? City sleep resembles an operating theater of lights, movement, and bleeping devices. We seek instant remedies for sleep, as for everything else. Of course, I am not going to give up alcohol, but I will throw in an herbal tea at the end of the evening. And I know to close the day with a book, although every few paragraphs my hand slides toward my iPhone, just to check messages or Instagram. Sometimes I try to meditate for a few minutes, which only jolts my memory of the emails I should have sent. This is not the path to the dreamless and perfect sleep of which Patrick Leigh Fermor writes.

The day after I had picked the book up, I happened to bump into my friend Tom Bradby, the ITV news anchor who had been off work for many months, suffering from extreme insomnia. He had recovered but had not forgotten his state or the causes of it. He had a new awareness of the meaning of what he called "the worried mind."

I reflected again on what Patrick Leigh Fermor had written: "In spite of private limitations, I was profoundly affected [by the monasteries]."

This was how I felt about my Norfolk ruins. I knew they touched me deeply but did not know why and certainly did not attribute it to any virtue on my part.

There is a wisdom in the monasteries that answers the affliction of our times. Renouncing the world, the monks and nuns have acquired a hidden knowledge of how to live. They labor, they learn, and they master what is described as "the interior silence." Some orders are in permanent retreat, but others are expected to maintain the stillness of self in the midst of public bustle. How can they do that? Is the virtue of interior silence something that can prevail in an era of peak technological distraction?

I was beginning to question my 5G life. The connectivity, the drip feed of news, the superficiality of politics. In the middle of the *Today* program, there is a three-and-a-half minute sermon by a religious figure. It is a peculiar anomaly in a daily news program, and many atheists have protested over the years, sometimes holding polite banners outside the BBC offices. But I have come to appreciate its situation. It is an oasis of reflection. News counts but meaning matters more.

I experienced that juxtaposition of connectivity and meaning at a dinner for the tech industry in the same week that I had read Patrick Leigh Fermor's book from cover to cover— properly read it, rather than speed-read it as I usually would.

I was satisfied that I had managed to cram in two social events before the dinner, traveling in a work version of the triathlon, by tube, bike, and foot. Never mind that I managed only to wave at a couple whom I had not seen for a long time. Whatever had happened in their lives in the past couple of years, I did not have the time to hear about it. At the second event I queued to sign in and then immediately turned and left. I was content with this level of productivity. I planned to give myself an hour and forty minutes at the dinner, before making the nightly late call to the office to check how much had changed in the world in that precise hour and forty minutes.

But the dinner's setting stopped me in my tracks. It was Lambeth Palace, seat of the archbishop of Canterbury. An artery road separates the palace from the river and the view of Parliament across the bridge. It is the wrong stretch of the wrong side of London. And yet behind the wall, hidden from the polluting traffic, is a garden second only to Buckingham Palace's, and a library that has the largest collection of religious books outside the Vatican.

I walked into the hall half-full with mostly male, mostly open-shirted entrepreneurs; progress assembled in human form. I talked to a fintech guy from Nigeria, to the creator of Alexa, to the inventor of Wikipedia, to the founder of Carphone Warehouse. The speaker, a cabinet minister, dryly explained to the room that the objects around the edge of the great hall were called books. We moved to a fashionably decorated tent in the garden for dinner. Many guests were checking their phones.

Then the archbishop of Canterbury, Justin Welby, arrived to welcome the slightly nonplussed room. It was, after all, his home. He had worked in the City in a previous life. He talked of the importance of connectivity in places such as Africa. Then he said that he hoped people would not find it awkward if he said a prayer. This was not a natural congregation, so the archbishop of Canterbury made a concession. He said for those who did not share his faith a contemplative silence would do. Some guests gingerly put down their phones at this point. There was not hush but silence. All you could hear was birdsong.

It was a moment of calmness before everyone struck up again. I longed for that calm.

I found a quote from R. S. Thomas, the Welsh poet and Anglican priest: "But the silence of the mind is when we live best."

I could not explain its meaning but I understood its significance.

And I recognized his description of the opposite state, a mind filled with noise, chaos, and anxiety. The modern condition.

The conversation at the tech gathering was all about pace of change and personal realization. We are driven by multiples of success and scale. Meanwhile, at my table, a broadcaster was looking furiously at her Twitter feed because a political joke she had made had started a bush fire of condemnation. By the end of the evening, her resignation from the BBC was being demanded. This was a time of maximum hubris, before the arrival of the great reckoning.

What if I were able to step away, even in the midst of political and media battle? There is a history of spiritual retreat after all.

"Attentiveness is the heart's stillness, unbroken by any thought," said Hesychius of Sinai. It is only when you stop, when you lay down your phone, that you can hear the birdsong.

In the Middle Ages, solitude and contemplation were regarded as necessary for enlightened living. The monasteries were admired as places of scholarship and spiritual ascent. The historian Tom Holland writes in his book *Dominion*:

> *Throughout Christian history, the yearning to reject a corrupt and contaminated world, to refuse any compromise with it, to aspire to a condition of untainted purity, would repeatedly manifest itself.*

If repeated through history, it must be an innate impulse. There is the world that we know and cannot challenge, except through laws, governments, or revolution. But some can live outside it, according to different rules.

The former Conservative strategist Lynton Crosby, who campaigned for Boris Johnson as mayor and later as prime minister, said to me that people were motivated by jobs, money, and family. His candidates won, he said, because he and they understood this.

The remarkable thing about the monasteries is that they are inspired by none of these things. They are there on behalf of humanity, suspended between heaven and earth. Some, of course, have fallen beneath the spheres. The number of monks is dropping. In Britain, the taint of abuse at the great monastic schools of Downside and Ampleforth has put off potential pupils and monks.

Yet the yearning for those original monastic values has not disappeared. The tranquil message of my Marham Abbey ruins and the great Rievaulx is humility. Personal ambition is an impediment, not a triumphant force.

There is an architectural reason for the monasteries' serenity, even when in ruins. They were laid out on an east-west axis, considered a calming alignment. The cloister had two elements, the garden open to the sky and the cloister passage, to allow the procession of monks with their holy water. Monasteries were also built near water and had superior drainage systems— another good reason for peace of mind.

There is something about the melancholy ruins against a Norfolk sky that reminds you that a contemplative life has a natural setting and that the endless striving and building around it will not last.

A monk, who once complained to an abbot at Rievaulx that he could not sleep, was advised to imagine that he was already in the grave.

For monks, death was the ultimate solace. Ignatius Loyola, a sixteenth-century Spanish priest who founded the Jesuits, had no doubt that death was a state of bliss. He contracted malaria, which was to prove fatal, in 1556, but he had been ready for this end for years. His followers wrote:

> *Thinking about death at this time he had such grand joy and such great spiritual consolation at being due to die that he was melting totally into tears. And this came to be such a recurring thing that he often used to refrain from thinking about death so as not to have so much of that consolation.*

Acceptance of death is something the world must learn anew. The enlightenment that makes the path between life and death one of aconites, snowdrops, and bluebells requires the greatest effort but also provides the greatest reward.

The early monastic letters of Saint Basil of Caesarea, who lived in the desert in the fourth century, used three epithets to describe his existence: light, peace, and happiness. How can we apply these principles to our worldly lives?

This is the chasm I am trying to close.

The monastic life demands an utterly different approach to the world. The Buddhist monk Gelong Thubten, who popularized the quest for profound happiness in his book *A Monk's*

Guide to Happiness, spent four years at a retreat on the Isle of Arran in Scotland. No phones, no internet, no newspapers. Twelve hours' meditation a day.

He wrote:

> *I remember thinking it was like having open-heart surgery with no anesthetic: You're backed into a corner with your most painful thoughts and feelings, with no distraction or escape.*

He mastered it, but while he was away he missed leaps of technology. The first thing he noticed on emerging from the retreat was the speed of things: "Everything and everyone moved so fast. Walking through London, I felt as if I had landed in a zombie apocalypse."

These are two worlds. The great difference between monastic joy and ours is that we depend on external gratification rather than inward happiness—which Thubten describes as freedom.

As Thubten wrote: "We live in a culture of doing rather than being."

Many have sought a solution in mindfulness but there is a crucial difference. Mindfulness does not help us escape our fight-or-flight existence—that demands a different state of being; a move from appetite, envy, and anxiety to compassion and appreciation.

I am searching for the remedy to our digital age. I cannot live the experience of Gelong Thubten, but I can explore this parallel existence and see if I can bring back something to my own life.

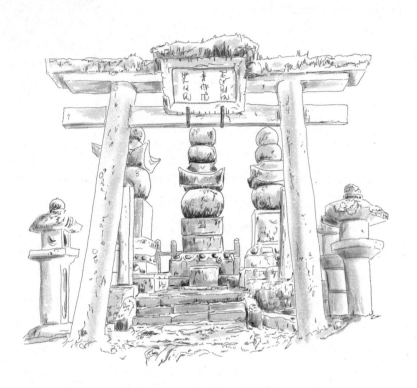

Chapter 1

HARMONY

KOYASAN, JAPAN

A friend of mine, named Thore Graepel, is a research scientist at Google's DeepMind. This puts him at the frontier of artificial intelligence; he is a student of the life of the mind. For him, humanity is still greater than the machine. The mind is naturally a polymath: It can respond to so many different things. Thore says: "Specialization is for insects." Understanding the mind is a formidable task; controlling it, the mission of monks. The question that people ask of Thore and his colleagues who work on AI is whether they are playing God. Yet there is nothing hubristic or arrogant about Thore. He has rather a shy manner, waiting for others to speak first. Neither does he have the unsocialized, garage-and-pizza persona we might associate with Silicon Valley scientists. Thore, who is from Germany but is now a British citizen, is homey. Family life is at the center of his Cambridge home. There is nothing virtual about the scene of bicycles in the hall, warm quiche fresh from the oven cooked by his wife, Susanne, and the immaculately stocked man shed.

Machine learning, Thore explains, progresses through experience rather than rules. It is trying to emulate a human mind, which is complex and unpredictable. We find it hard to describe and explain our thought processes. Our minds can at times become a bit of a jumble. We jump from one thought to another. The iPhone mind is a condition of our age. We scroll rather than settle. And we have no way of ordering the mass of information invading our minds. It is just piles of stuff, everywhere.

Thore is a leading research scientist, but he is also a Buddhist. His children point to the portrait of Enlightenment on the wall showing the ten stages of meditation—depicted as a monk's journey with a dark elephant and a monkey, representing hindrance and distraction. There are flames representing effort, which disappear as the ease of meditation triumphs. The angry elephant turns white and placid until it is ridden by the monk. The monkey vanishes. What has taken place is an uncluttering of the mind.

Thore explains that meditation is as necessary to him as AI. His work in AI is physical and cognitive, a discipline for understanding the mind. It concerns itself with the architecture of the brain. Meditation comes from within; it is not intellectual but intuitive. Both physics and meditation demand sustained training. Thore claims that Buddhist meditation is a kind of science—a contemplative science, evidence based and empirical. Buddha is a teacher who said "find out for yourself"—just as Galileo did.

But science and meditation have different outcomes. It is the second which concerns us in this chapter. It is a sort of baptism of the mind, through cleansing.

I once went to the banks of the River Jordan to watch the Christian baptisms take place. Here the pilgrims come in their buses, along barricaded and border-controlled roads—the environment of conflict—to reach the banks of the brownish, swollen river. Men and women, old and young, wade into the middle to be dunked in the biblical waters. It is the greatest public act of faith, photographed, applauded. One young woman I watched was so overcome by the experience that afterward she was shaking in her thin summer dress, not cold, but momentarily transformed. The transformation is an ascension from the weight of human clutter to a purified state.

As Thomas Carlyle wrote:

Thou there, the thing for thee to do is, if possible, to cease to be a hollow sounding shell of hearsays, egoisms, purblind dilettantisms; and become, were it on the infinitely small scale, a faithful discerning soul.

The cleansing of the mind is a different kind of baptism; quiet, minimalist, internal.

There is no public confirmation, for who knows what is inside man other than the Lord?

The challenge is that the mind can seem like merely a series of sensations. How do you control the inner dialogue? Thore says that he had heard of a CEO who claimed to have cognitive control of his inner thoughts at work, but this was unusual. The rest of us need periods of concentration and years of practice to achieve peace of mind.

The standard textbook for the ten stages of meditation is called *The Mind Illuminated*, by Matthew Immergut and a former neuroscience professor, now Buddhist instructor, named Culadasa. Here are the first five stages:

First: Establish a daily practice, building up from fifteen minutes a day.

Second: Practice the hard and continuous training of stopping the mind from wandering.

Third: Extend the periods of concentration.

Fourth: Overcome dullness. This generally means stopping yourself from falling asleep, but encompasses a lack of "peripheral awareness." Your mind should be still but attentive, rather than drowsy.

Fifth: Increase mindfulness. This is the start of the process of unifying the mind.

By stage eight, the senses are pacified, by nine you should be entering meditative joy, and by ten enjoying a state of tranquility and equanimity.

A handbook on peace of mind, in ten stages.

As with physics or playing the piano, I realize illuminating my mind is going to take time and attention. Effortlessness is hard. Culadasa uses the words *diligence*, *vigilance*, and *effort* to describe what is required to reach this state of bliss. I confess that, since sleep deprivation is a professional issue for me, I quite like dullness. I meditate in order to fall asleep.

I decide to follow the instructions in the book, though my quest is not mindfulness but the secrets of monasticism. I want to unclutter my mind. I am looking for order, harmony, and ceremony to counter the chaotic, unsifted news cycle of my life. After some research, I realize that the form of monasticism that answers this need is Japanese Temple Buddhism.

If I think of Japan, it is of Tokyo. It is the nearest thing I know to London: It is built on its work ethic. When I edited a London newspaper, I asked research groups to test reactions to certain words on the front page. Which words would persuade readers to pick up the newspaper? I knew for instance that the word *family* was attractive to readers of the *Daily Mail* and *pension* was of immediate interest for readers of the *Daily Telegraph*. The words that caught the eye of *Evening Standard* readers— apart from names of celebrities and unexpected deaths—were *jobs* and *bonuses*.

The stillness of monasticism is antithetical to news and the baubles and babble of cities. Far away from Tokyo are temple monasteries clustered around mountains, where the air is clear and the views are silhouettes of peaks and shrubs and clouds in the shapes of lily pads, shot through with promise or memory of sunlight. One lesson of monasticism is leaving behind the familiar. Japan takes me from West to East. And there is another layer of unfamiliarity, which is the vibrant interplay of materialism and spiritualism. A characteristic of Japanese monasticism is that it exists within society. The monks can marry and have children. They are distinctive through their shaved heads and their robes, but otherwise you will see them at railway stations or in shops, in the swim of humanity. And yet they have a core of separateness. How can I find the secret of that coexistence? The inner nun.

● ● ●

Serendipitously, I already have a plan to go to Japan because the *Today* program is broadcasting from there ahead of the G20 economic summit. In 2019 I start to look up routes and connections online. I could take the train from Tokyo to an unfamiliar landscape, language, culture, faith—to the monasteries of Koyasan, south of Osaka, a land of spiritual dreams.

I have another desire, removed from professional life. I want to renew empathy with my twenty-four-year-old daughter. She is urban, clever, and impatient for social justice. She finds my life too politically complacent. This has been a year of Brexit turmoil, old against young, rural against cities, Leave against Remain.

Relationships require attention; you can't keep half an ear out for them. Fortunately, my daughter and I share a common aspiration that can draw us together: We are both seeking equilibrium among these opposites. We both want peace of mind. The bridge between us is love. The challenge is minimalism. We have to slough off our prejudices, our positions, and most of all our possessions.

My hoarding takes a particular form. It is basically books and toiletries. I have always thought that makeup and toiletries are the material comforts that are just below the guilt line of extravagance. I can happily shop without buying clothes. But I always linger over a newly packaged moisturizer or bath oil.

When my daughter's boyfriend stayed overnight at our London home, he was aghast at the pharmacy that had colonized the bathroom, at the different brands of cleansers, not always finished, because my eye had fastened on something freshly tempting. Day creams and night creams and serums and hand creams spread beyond cabinets to windowsills. To me, it was a menagerie; to my daughter's boyfriend, the hoarding of Miss Havisham.

I saw a documentary about a community of nuns in the South of England in which a novice confessed that her greatest self-doubt was whether she could give up her array of toiletries. She made the leap. I honestly don't think I ever could. Monasticism allows small pleasures: wine or honey. But material comforts are at odds with it.

For reasons of climate and inequality, my daughter has turned her back on materialism and buys her clothes from charity shops. But that does not stop her from opening the bathroom cabinet as if it were the bell-ringing door of a sweet shop. Our mother-daughter bonding hovers between books and mani-pedis, seriousness and frivolity.

As I am packing in between evening calls and emails, I receive a GIF WhatsApp message from my daughter. It is a storybook picture from Beatrix Potter, of a mother rabbit in starched cotton and apron handing a mug of milk to a child rabbit in a wooden bed with plumped-up pillow and billowing duvet. Her caption reads: "Goodnight mama."

My independent daughter sends the message in a spirit of laughing irony, but it strikes my heart. I wish I could express my love for her through simple maternal gestures. I crave intimacy.

I reply with a quote from Saint Augustine: "The world is a book and those who do not travel read only one page." Then I phone her to say that I am leaving for Japan and want her to join me. Could we just leave everything behind and go? To my delight, my daughter says: "Yes."

My daughter agreeing to join me isn't exactly Peter the disciple, giving up everything in an act of faith, but it exhibits a carefree spirit that I am thrilled to share. I have been so hemmed in by work commitments I have missed out on emotional experiences. I have loved my daughter all her life, but how well do I know her?

Pilgrims travel light. We dare each other into tiny luggage. She a small rucksack, me a shoulder bag, heavy only with books. We do not need stuff.

There are two Buddhist scholars in Japan who exercise the greatest influence: Saicho and Kobo Daishi, and their rivalry continues, more than a thousand years later. I would say a thousand years after their deaths, but this contradicts a central claim of eternal meditation, that death is not a separate state.

Saicho is associated with the Chinese coastal strain of Tendai Buddhism. His philosophy is based on service. His mantra is "Forget self and benefit others." *Forget self* seems to me the secret password to peace of mind. Saicho also advised perpetual wonder and gratitude for being alive and human. Consumerism and individualism dull this sense of joy. Our roots, he said, must stay firmly in the "tree of family."

The word *harmony* appears often in descriptions of Tendai Buddhism. Harmony with nature, harmony with fellow men. The word still resonates in Japan. The new emperor Naruhito, who succeeded his father in May 2019, has his own imperial era, which is called Reiwa. It means beautiful harmony.

The word is used with ease by politicians and business people in a way that sounds comically odd to a British ear. Before going to Koyasan, I meet the president of Fujitsu in Tokyo. He describes his role as bringing harmony and happiness to the public. At another function, a student says that she hopes her future in management consultancy will bring about a more harmonious world. I raise my eyebrows and grin at the translator and she asks: "Do business people not talk like this in Britain?"

Perhaps we are too cynical, or maybe our language is simply not constructed around concepts such as societal happiness and virtue. We talk of individual fulfillment, but this tends to be linked to a commitment to self. I believe that my spirit will become clearer if I lose this burdensome sense of self.

My twin aims, then, are to learn how to subdue my mind and to find a harmony with my daughter. The legend of Koyasan is potent. It claims this isolated place of mountains and rivers was consecrated by the great Buddhist teacher Kobo Daishi in AD 819.

In the legend, Kobo Daishi, traveling back to Japan from China where he'd been studying Buddhism, prayed for help to find the perfect place to build a monastery. As part of his prayer, he threw a triple-forked vajra (a mythical weapon) into the sea, in the direction of Japan.

Once back on home soil, Kobo Daishi set off for the mountains, where he encountered a huntsman and two dogs. The huntsman indicated a mysterious light that hung over Mount Koya, and then vanished.

Kobo Daishi followed the bright light between the trees all the way to Koyasan, and there found a pine tree with the triple-forked vajra lodged in it.

The teaching of Kobo Daishi is that enlightenment can be achieved within a lifetime. "If one maintains the mind of the Buddha while searching for the Buddha's wisdom, then one can become a Buddha in this very existence." According to legend, Kobo Daishi took on the form of the great Sun Buddha, pouring out light.

The education of the monks of Koyasan was designed by Kobo Daishi. It covered Buddhism, Confucianism, Taoism, law, logic, diplomacy, music, horsemanship, calligraphy, mathematics, grammar, medicine, art, philosophy, and astronomy. These were the subjects that he believed were necessary for intellectual and spiritual enlightenment. Kobo Daishi believed in the health of the body, mind, and spirit.

My daughter and I travel separately because she has things to do. I look out from the plane window, reminded of Georgia O'Keeffe's painting *Sky Above Clouds*. The multiplying flat, white clouds on a blue surface resemble infinity. They are serenely beyond the world's surface. I think of my daughter traveling at the same speed and distance just behind me. My flight from London is at 7:15 P.M. Wednesday, arriving at 3:00 P.M. Thursday, into Haneda Airport. The trick is to find my daughter, who has left at midday on Wednesday via Hong Kong, from where she is taking a connecting flight.

We agree to meet at the Wi-Fi stall, to collect pocket Wi-Fi for maximum connectivity. I think: "What if her phone battery is dead and I actually can't find her?" I have the tense, searching face of someone who has a rational assumption that all will be well but an imaginative fear that it will not. The face of a parent in other words.

There she is: The familiar easy stride, long back, taller than me, hair behind her ears; she slings an arm around my neck. She smells of youth and travel. Although she has been flying for more than twenty-four hours, she is ready to push on. We follow the arrows along the station to the bullet train; I chide her about using her phone and then see she has worked out times and routes on the internet more effectively than I have trying to read signs on the platform.

Life experience has been superseded by tech savvy. I send her to get the Rail Passes as if it is a test of responsibility, when in fact it saves me the humiliation of failing to speak the language.

We take the express train and then the bullet train to Kyoto. I am feeling neither calm nor selfless, fretting about having bought the wrong kind of phone charger, passive-aggressively blaming my daughter for not noticing that I had, anxious that the train connections are too tight. My daughter's head tilts onto my shoulder and her eyelids close. I smooth her tangled airplane hair, my fretfulness mingled with fondness.

There is a poise to the other passengers—commuters and students—opposite us. They don't spread out in the way they do in London. Their heads are upright. Outside the cabin-style windows is the flash of construction: high buildings, cranes, and bright lights. We get off the train, dash across two subways, my daughter checking her phone, me glancing at the weal on my forearm from the strap of my bag. I feel a childish, tired self-pity. My daughter shrugs impatiently—she is developing a Southeast Asian sensibility—and runs ahead to the central station.

We have made it, and in the midevening we reach the pleasantly ordered former imperial city of Kyoto. We find a hotel and a restaurant of wood and glass; there is symmetry and order. Both the menu and the waitress give directions in Japanese so my order is a stab in the dark and my daughter and I are united in laughter. That night, I sleep fitfully as if still on the plane and wake to find my phone is dead. We think, "It does not matter, we are in a major Japanese city." We stroll down the main street, looking at cute pug dogs and gadgets in the windows, and peering into coffee shops. There are no adapters.

And then it is back to the station. And I am biting my nails as I look at my dead phone. The first train takes about thirty minutes; we leg it to change to the second, about fifteen more minutes, then change again, and again. Onward, onward. The trains run on time and time runs on. We are pure motion. In Japan, even the rain is contained in box-like bursts of about fifteen minutes.

On the final train from Hashimoto to Gokurakubashi station, the scenery changes and so does the weather. A heavy shower has ritually cleansed the already-green hills and foliage. The train line would delight any Hornby collector, its clean little stations, with their troughs of bright flowers on the narrow platforms and their merry signs carved into the mountain.

The train winds through banks of bamboo trees on one side and mountains and valleys on the other. Woods, deep ravines, a clear river running over smooth stones. At Gokurakubashi station—Mrs. Tiggy-winkle clean and tidy—a cable car is waiting to haul us up to Koyasan. An alternative route is to take the path over a painted footbridge named Bridge to Paradise.

I should not have worried about the train connections. Everything here runs like clockwork. But now I want to learn a monastic sense of time, a sense of purpose and rhythm without the days feeling crammed. I am trying to train myself out of the silos of the West. I want to learn to be still without succumbing to boredom.

The only other passengers in the cable car are a couple in their thirties, male and female, Southern Hemisphere, athletic, a tenderness of glances and smiles between them. He is reading Kazuo Ishiguro. They are basking in a different kind of relationship with Japanese monasticism.

Mine stretches across a generation, and different perspectives. It is a journey of recovered memories, regrets, letting go, and reuniting. For them, it is the joy of discovery of each other.

The cable car lurches us up through ferns and lichen-covered woodland to a pristine village of Swiss-style wooden houses with pagoda roofs. Among the monks here are little bands of foreign pilgrims. The "Buddhist tourists" tend to come in their droves in spring or autumn, for the cherry blossom and the maple trees. But it is midsummer, so there are no crowds now.

Cherry blossom is celebrated across Japan, but there are two particular ancient cherry trees here, recorded by the twelfth-century Japanese poet Saigyo. He left his wife, children, and the army to become a wandering poet. This was his will:

This is my wish
That under the cover of the blossom

I may die in spring,
That day of the second month,
Just when the moon is full.

Aboard the mountain bus, we follow the weight of the greenery thinning into a clearing. Here at last is the mountain monastery, its topography forming a lotus flower with eight peaks for petals. Mountain and monastery, the conditions of harmony.

There are two symbols that express the land of Koyasan. The first is the Bell of the Daito: the sound of the mountain, the voice of the Buddha. It rings more than one hundred times a day to liberate those within hearing from the evil passions of living. The second is the lotus pond. The lotus reminds us that nature is pure and that we can obtain peace of mind. It would be a baptism for me to incorporate bells and lotus ponds into my existence. But I am not there yet.

The bus takes us to the gates of the guest lodgings. They are made of heavy carved wood and iron, with a rope of straw—not a partition but a step into a different world. In the early evening the monks are preparing for the night. We dip our heads to step through into a courtyard. At the center of the square is an old mulberry tree. A monk is reading by it. We bow and take the steps up to the wooden terrace of the guesthouse. Lanterns hang in lines from the roof: the divine light. All shoes are neatly laid here and we add our own. A monk greets us, with barely any movement, and leads us down polished wooden corridors until we reach our room. It is empty but for a low table with two floor chairs. Sliding screen doors open to a little inner courtyard surrounded by trees. The monk opens the cupboard to show futon beds, which are taken out at night.

Our little bags look messy and overstuffed, and the monk appears momentarily pained as I start to scatter contents onto the floor. I immediately vow to pare down my existence further. I think guiltily of rooms back home; drawers crammed with a mix of favored and discarded clothes, papers and books piled up, every surface a dumping ground.

The chaos of my handbag resembles the disorder of my mind, I realize. One thing I will learn from this place is that tidiness is a condition of harmony. When I check outside the door, I notice that the slippers that were lent to me, and which I left askew on the doorstep, have been straightened. Trainee monks are taught a foreign language—and how to be clean and tidy.

For minds to be clear, surroundings should be simple. The attraction of the monasteries is the lack of distraction, of appetite, of excess.

We eat at six; Buddhist vegetarian dishes based on the concept of five flavors, five cooking methods, and five colors. A meal should include something grilled, something deep-fried, some thing pickled, tofu, and soup. We try sushi, dried plum, udo, yam, lotus root, snow peas, nori seaweed, water shield, powder pepper. It is both filling and cleansing. But I cannot find a way of sitting comfortably in the Buddhist style. I kneel, then sag onto one side, then try an inflexibly tight cross-legged position, then return to kneeling. My daughter is agile and graceful. The physicality of meditation is not something I had thought about.

After our feast, which somehow avoided gluttony, we walk in the soft half-light around the temple area before getting back through our little wooden door in time for the curfew. A gong sounds at 9:00 P.M. The monks rise in time for 6:00 A.M. prayers. Early to bed and early to rise is not just a homily but at the root of monasticism.

The little pillow is stuffed with rice or what feels like small stones. My head makes an indentation, but this is not a princess pillow. As for the mattress on the floor, it does not suit my normal fetal position, so I arrive by the lack of options at the correct posture, lying on my back, arms by my side. There is darkness and silence. Yet I sleep terribly, mostly because of the time difference, but also because my mind races with looped worries that I am low on Japanese currency and I have not yet found a charger and what must we do tomorrow, and what on earth is happening in the office and in emails and on Twitter. And my dreams are of organizing events that go awry and of being in the wrong place. A passage from Matthew's Gospel runs through my head: "Look at the birds of the air, for they neither sow nor reap nor gather into barns; yet your heavenly Father feeds them."

I should think less chaotically, although it has to be said I have had some good ideas among the maelstrom, including one for a career change after the *Today* program. I decide that next summer I will leave my job. Serenity comes with the realization that I have no plan. Rather than enforcing my will on myself and others, I will see what happens. I shall float on the surface like the lotus pads.

It is quite different waking to an empty room. The mattress that had felt skimpy when I lay down feels sufficient in the morning. The closeness to the floor gives a sense of gravity, the lack of a soft pillow stretches out the body. Beyond the shape of my daughter's beloved head laid sideways under the duvet is the open screen door and light piercing the thin wall beyond it.

Just before six I rise without waking my daughter—monasticism has taught me to move softly—to find the prayer room. There are four rows of chairs in front of an altar. It is decorated in reds and gold and the candles are lit. Three monks appear from side entrances, and the service begins. They bow low, and slide a string of beads through their hands. They pick up prayer books, and the low incantatory chanting starts. I do not know what they are saying, but my thoughts become less crowded and I am lulled by the chants.

In the catechism—translated by Philip Nicoloff in his book *Sacred Kōyasan*—the monks tell the story of the Cosmic Buddha taking his place in the highest heavens. Appetites are named; male appetites of lust and sovereignty, female appetites of craving and pride. The cheerful news is that these can be overcome. Then the monks address the "three poisons"—greed, hate, and delusion.

Esoteric Buddhism preaches transformation rather than eradication. The message ends in conformation. The essence of humanity is good. The final prayer:

> *We wish that the vow of enlightenment never cease, guiding all beings equally toward the attainment of the ultimate world— and that we may all enter together into the land of the Buddha Dainichi, for it is His nature that we share.*

When they finish, the congregation—a handful of pilgrims and observers like me—is invited to sit at a stall and take flakes from a bowl on the right, scattering them onto a bowl of smoking incense and a kind of broth on the left. The service comes to an end and I return to my room. At 7:01 A.M. the phone rings and a monk tells us we are late for 7:00 breakfast. Strict timekeeping I admire and intend to copy. As a journalist, I observe punctuality because lateness can mean losing the story or the interview. I am now learning about timekeeping for its own sake. With routine, with order, will come sleep.

Breakfast is soup and Japanese vegetables and tea. I experience a weary longing for a chocolate croissant and cappuccino, my usual breakfast. If I am to learn peace of mind, I must be broken down to be remade, starting with my diet. I whisper to my daughter: "Wouldn't you love a takeaway coffee now?" She rolls her eyes and shakes her head. I have brought her to Koyasan in a junior role. Yet so far, I am the one with a busted phone and clinging to London habits. She is a lotus flower by comparison. As for the phone, she has a word with one of the monks, and returns with a charger in her hand. I say: "Oh no, now I shall have to look at Twitter."

But then I choose not to. And I immediately start to feel less fretful. Nobu, a local monk, arrives at 9:00 A.M., to show us around.

We follow him in a straight line along the road to look at the main Kongobuji Temple. Before entering, we ritually cleanse our hands, ladling water onto each and bringing a splash of it to our mouths. Cleanliness is valued highly. Cleanliness on the outside is equated to cleanliness within. Well, we can start there. There are gaps within the temple corridors for little gardens, which we explore. I study the Zen garden. My garden at home in Norfolk is a merry chaos of color and season. Outside my window, wild roses fight with lilac and clematis. By contrast, the Zen garden is a collection of aligned granite rocks laid on mossy grass. It calms rather than excites. Order trumps passion.

The next garden, the Shingon-shu, is a varied cluster of trees and shrubs of different heights. Biodiversity is Buddhist: everyone different, in one community. We stop to read some calligraphy on a wall, a quote from Kobo Daishi: "Do not talk about the failings of others or your own virtues." I am feeling more at home here, in a place about as conceptually distanced from the world of media as possible.

We walk on, in sunshine cooled by crisp mountain air, to the Dango Garan sacred temple complex. The fundamental pagoda, the Great Stupa, is painted the color of fire, and had clearly been a victim of it in the past. Within is the Cosmic Buddha, representing the universe, with hands in womb position. There are other Buddhas here too, including the Medicine Buddha, the first to be created by monks. Monks medicine is the founding principle of this Buddha. It is the basic need of humanity. Where there are monks, there is medicine, education, and consolation. A piece of script nearby reminds us that color is void and void is color. All is impermanent. Make the most of the life that you have. This is the particular teaching of Kobo Daishi. Do not wait for another life; this is the one to get right.

We stop among the cedars and the cypresses to look at a board hung with messages written on pieces of wood. The wishes of the people conform around the world: They ask for good health, for a happy family. In Japan, the added fervent wish is for success in exams.

The symmetry of male-dominated wisdom and female-dominated compassion is believed to be the route to enlightenment. Yet women were not permitted on this mountain until the nineteenth century. The reason given was that women would distract the young monks and that the lady god would be jealous of other women. "There goes the patriarchy again, trying to turn women against women," says my daughter scornfully. We have generationally different levels of expectations on female rights. I have operated on the principle that it is off-putting to go on about it too much. When I was my daughter's age, I valued the aberration of female achievement and regarded the first female prime minister of the UK, Margaret Thatcher, as if she were a brilliant explorer.

My daughter demands the same rights for all women and regards Margaret Thatcher as insufficiently sisterly; even less forgivable, she was Conservative. We usually get round this by avoiding the subject, but today my daughter has me within her sights. Over a weak coffee in the village, she lectures me on the legacy of damage that Mrs. Thatcher has caused, on my misplaced faith in hard work being the only answer to everything, on my narrow privilege. I try to change the subject, but my daughter is an English graduate and knows how to trap an opponent in rhetoric. I tell her that I am increasingly valuing the gift of silence.

When we continue our walk, it is at a greater physical distance from each other. I wonder if monks argue with each other. Women may not have been welcomed as worshippers on this mountain, but women were worshipped. Rather like the relationship between women in the Conservative Party and Margaret Thatcher, my daughter might say.

On the right of Dainichi Buddha is the goddess Benten, the central deity of Esoteric Buddhism, associated with the Indian river goddess Sarasvati. There are several shrines to Benten in Koyasan, for she is the goddess of "flowing things," of river and valley.

Another figure revered here is En the Ascetic, a seventh-century mountain mystic whose sheer self-discipline gave him the power of flight. In *Sacred Kōyasan*, Philip Nicoloff cites a legend that En was finally so enlightened that he put his mother in a Buddhist alms bowl and flew off to China with her, where they achieved immortality. Every woman with a son must sigh contentedly over that image. I am missing my less-critical two sons. I make a note to try to include them in future monastic experiences.

My daughter and I find a way out of our confrontation. Sometimes it is better to stand on ceremony. It binds us into a civility of form. The answer to our scratchiness is a tea ceremony. This, like everything else here, is a spiritual lesson. It is about acquiring discipline.

Our tea master demonstrates the tender intricacy of the ceremony. The wiping of the cup and the display of its less-worn side to guests. The swilling of hot water. The exact amount of green powder on the spoons. The flourish of the dried grass whisk to get the right consistency. The smallness of gestures. Mine by contrast looks like watery watercress soup. The sins of carelessness and impatience revealed. My daughter tries harder and does better. We are getting on famously, encouraging each other's efforts. We hold each other's gaze, smiling.

Next door is the meditation class. Outside, there are some frog-green lotus leaves in a large black bowl of water, placed next to a granite rock. I look at it with a rush of pleasure. Here I am with the daughter I love, breathing mountain air, looking at lotus leaves. My phone throbs in my pocket with a news update. I shudder and turn it off. Our meditation teacher is sitting cross-legged on the polished wooden floor of the room, the window open. His eyes are shuttered, his mind controlled. He smiles and murmurs to us. Sit up straight, breathe deeply, in and out, eyes half-closed, balanced between visibility and invisibility, the external and the internal. If you can control your breath, you can control your mind. Mine is still jittery from events of the day, but at last I am starting to slow down. And I am content.

As Kobo Daishi said: "It is even possible for a fool to practice asceticism, by way of temperance in eating and self-reproach. He is delighted who is content with little, and learns and practices often."

In the early evening, my daughter and I step out of the monastery gates again; we are going to the forest cemetery to look at the mausoleum of Kobo Daishi. As dusk falls, we meld like shadows into a larger group of people walking as one. It feels more like an orchestra than a crowd. We are in tune with each other. As the light fades, the tall Japanese cedar trees close in on us, Tolkien-style. My daughter walks up to one of them and circles it with her arms. Close up, the bark is layered and warm as if it is breathing. Its roots spread across the ground like plaited ropes of hair. Along the path, shrines repeat the image of the moon, a symbol of enlightenment. I understand that this forest walk is a kind of communion. Despite the swelling congregation of walkers, we make no imprint on the earth; we are here, then gone.

"When you tremble with worry, contemplate the truth that all elements of this world are nonsubstantial and impermanent." (Kobo Daishi)

Our monk moves easily among the shrines; there is a closer relationship between the living and the dead in this part of Japan. Ancestors are friends.

Before we reach the mausoleum, we are meant to wash in the river, but because it is now black night, with only the light of the stars sparkling above the pillars of the trees, we instead splash the Buddha statues with river water. We then bow, before walking to the gates of the mausoleum. Its height and decoration are splendid even in darkness. This is the Temple of the Dragon Light. Within is the room of Kobo Daishi's entrance into continual meditation.

It was in AD 831, when Kobo Daishi was fifty-eight, my age, that he prepared for death. He conducted a ceremony at Koyasan known as the offering ceremony of Ten Thousand Lights and Flowers and selected his burial place at the side of the valley, by a fast-flowing stream.

At midnight, he took his final breath. His watching disciples saw that his eyes closed, but there was no other change. He was still upright. No formal funeral was held because he appeared to be not dead but meditating.

The monk describes under his breath the history of the mausoleum of Kobo Daishi. Questions spring to mind: For instance, is he a skeleton? But this is a literal Western way of looking at things. Perhaps we should be more metaphorical. If enlightenment can be in the present, it is lasting. The story has obvious echoes of the resurrection of Jesus Christ.

I suddenly shiver with cold. I look round, at the shifting shape of my daughter, who takes my hand. The group starts to disperse, and I walk the soft tree-needle route alone with her. I ask if she has found it strange or frightening; walking among the dead. She says that to her it felt natural. We do not talk about death in the West, so we do not get our partings right. I will lose my parents, my daughter will lose me. In this soft forest earth it feels as if generations stretching back coexist, in life and death.

We sometimes find faith hard to pitch right, but I think my daughter and I understand here both the transience of humanity and its eternity in the infinite universe. Then, in the final stretch of the cemetery, the joy in creation sours. It is a wide boulevard with shrines in the shape of, among other things, giant cups and rocket engines. These are the corporate shrines, donated by companies to the ancestors of their workers. "Buying souls," my anti-capitalist daughter murmurs crossly. Politics has separated us again.

We just make the 9:00 P.M. curfew, return to our rooms, fold our clothes neatly, and lie on our mattresses. We make barely any mess or noise. My daughter soon sleeps, her breathing even; I am awake but peaceful. I get up and slip out through the screen doors of our room into the courtyard. A giant cedar tree is silhouetted in my sight line and its reassuring presence makes me feel safe and drowsy.

The night air is both caressing and sharp. It is silent except for the occasional screech of a flying squirrel. I stand and pray to the mountain. Or rather, I give thanks, which is a kind of prayer. When I wake, eight hours later, the cedar tree is suffused with the early-morning light. The monks are heading for prayers. My daughter and I put our beds back in the cupboard and make sure the curtains are drawn symmetrically. Then we slip away to the sound of chanting.

When we leave, the monks of Koyasan give me a little book of sayings by Kobo Daishi to take with me. But the nature of the mountain, which is at the center of Kobo Daishi's monasticism, I must leave behind. Here are a few sayings I particularly like:

The lonely cloud has no path home and loves a distant peak.

I don't claim to know worldly things: I just watch the moon and lie down beneath a green pine.

In the end I've had no interest in momentary glories, in an imperial court or the markets.

My strongest desire is for the flowing fog on a mountain, and a marshy meadow in the morning and the evening.

I am softened by the experience of Koyasan but remain firmly in the first stage of enlightenment, appetite without ethics. I have in my hand the plug adapter, lent to me by the monks, and there is nobody to whom to return it at the entrance of the guesthouse. I make no effort to look for the monk. Knowing how hard I had found it to purchase one and the unlikelihood of getting one on the next stage of our journey, I keep it in my pocket, and pray for forgiveness.

Out of the dawn mist arrives the bus to the cable car, and our journey continues by train, then a second, third, and fourth train, in time to get passage to the island of Naoshima, or Art Island.

There is a car ferry and a passenger ferry over to the island, and seeing a stationary passenger ferry, we go and wait by it. A young European woman wanders over to us to ask where we get tickets and what time the ferry goes. My daughter helpfully consults her phone and directs the girl to the ticket office. Next thing, we see her running to the next dock to jump on what we now see is another passenger ferry, moments before it leaves.

My daughter watches her with indignation. "She could have told us! She knew that we were going on the passenger ferry." I draw on Kobo Daishi and tell her that the car ferry will be more fun. We pick our way through the fumes of the cars, finding our plastic seats on the upper deck.

The islands emerge from the sea like the rocks in the Zen garden. We are heading for the distant peak, and after an hour we reach the narrow sandy shore of Art Island. This is where art and nature combine, giving rise to a religious experience. There is public art everywhere, starting with the bright yellow pumpkin sculpture on the beach.

In Norfolk, I am a neighbor of the artist Antony Gormley, whose art depicts the religious experience of landscape. He sculpts figures, man alone facing the elements, the pilgrim in nature. At Art Island, the public works create art in relationship with nature. A yellow wooden rowing boat on the beach appears again in an art gallery in the interior of the island. The art is in the use of color and the position of the boat, among pebbles and grasses, between sea and sky. This is a serene place, a monastery of art.

We walk up the path to the top of the hill; the air is waterfall clear and smells of ferns and jasmine. We approach the Chichu Art Museum, just past a lily pond—the sacred lotus in pinks and reds, the bowing trees reflected in the water. Water lilies have a particular effect on me, especially now that I know them as lotus flowers. My great-great-grandfather James Hudson was head gardener for Leopold de Rothschild at Gunnersbury Park in London. A lily was named after him, the Nymphaea "James Hudson." Hudson created a garden in France, where he built a wooden bridge over a lily pond. It was a garden visited by the French painter Claude Monet. It is an ambition of my journey to dig a pond at my home in Norfolk and bring the Hudson lilies there.

We enter the gray concrete gallery as if into a mirror. Here are the paintings of Monet, the lily ponds outside reflected but also given enhanced beauty and depth. Monet has improved on nature.

In order to enter the Monet room, we are asked by attendants, dressed in white, to exchange shoes for slippers. There is a policy of no photographs, to encourage people to contemplate the art rather than record it with a selfie. It is as if one is entering a church. The religious experience continues in the room dedicated to the artist of light James Turrell. Only a few visitors at a time are permitted to ascend the steps toward a milky white light, so that you are within the light, as if in a cloud. Then a screen begins to change color, to a deepening blue, and when you turn back the steps at the entrance have turned rust red.

I am reminded again of Kobo Daishi: "The one who has attained Buddhahood is neither blue, yellow, red, white, vermillion, purple, clear, long, short, round, square, bright, dark, male, female, nor genderless." The beautiful transience of color in the James Turrell room creates a mystical experience. The self becomes abstract. There is no end and no beginning.

My daughter says that the Monet and the Turrell, in different ways, leave her both joyful and tearful.

We stroll back down the path, arms around each other, stopping to look at some more public art. A flexible steel arch stretches skyward between two rocks on a grassy bank. A steel mat beneath has a mirror effect. The arch frames the milky sea and the ships that glide across it.

A woman of middle years is taking small steps down to the arch installation and kneels down in front of it, looking out to sea. She is wearing a gray dress and a habit. She is a nun. The shape of her habit, the steel mirror mat in front of her, the lines of coast, and the ships beyond all form part of a greater natural portrait.

I think again of Koyasan and the dominating figure of the Cosmic Buddha representing the universe. What we are searching for is cosmic harmony. There is a glimpse of it here. Peace of the universe, peace of mind.

The morning light is like the screens in my Koyasan room— back-lit clouds, the sea like a sheet of metal, the line of ships heading for the China Sea cutting through it. We catch the passenger ferry, my daughter observing the European who had betrayed their social contract on the way over. She says, eyebrow arched, that she is prepared to forgive her, as Jesus forgave mankind. We sit side by side on a bench on the deck. Her T-shirt is warm from the sun when I hug her. We chug away from the contemplative island toward the mainland port.

My daughter heads off home while I stay on in Tokyo for work, the beauty of Koyasan and Art Island contained within us. Monasticism internalizes beauty and love. We have experienced harmony.

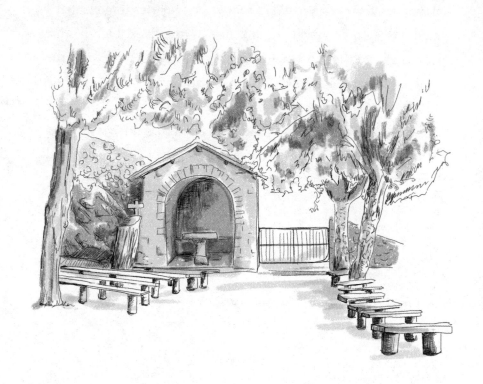

Chapter 2

SELF-DENIAL AND NATURE

FRANCIS OF ASSISI

n the week that Boris Johnson is elected prime minister, greeted by the president of the United States as "Britain's Trump," I am at the tomb of Francis of Assisi. I am drawn away from the billboard personalities of alpha males to the quiet of a thirteenth-century friar, who considered himself the lowliest of men and was regarded by pilgrims as Christ-like.

I have been to Assisi before. My former boss, the proprietor of the *Evening Standard*, Evgeny Lebedev, had a castle on a hill above the city. His weekend salons ferried guests between this fabulous castle near Perugia and his palazzo in Umbria.

It was my job as editor of the London newspaper to deliver Boris Johnson to these weekends. The preparations were elaborate, and our welcoming party would breathe more deeply when our cars finally accelerated up the avenue of cypresses, taking in the jasmine air, and preparing for a weekend of medieval splendor; feasting, dancing, boar hunting. I have a memory of a disheveled Johnson chasing Evgeny's wolf, also named Boris, because it had eaten his computer dongle.

Evgeny's castle was gorgeously attired, with the finest furniture, fabrics, and art—a mixture of religious, historical, and contemporary profane. It was the kind of home that would have been familiar to Francis of Assisi before his conversion. As a young man, Francis led a Perugian life. He was the son of a wealthy merchant; a knight and an aesthete. But he gave all this up for penitence and self-mortification.

I sense I am going to need a different approach for this chapter. My mission is to learn about monastic life from experience, or at least find ways of folding moments of monasticism into my life. Saint Francis is much more demanding. Like Jesus, he gave up everything.

I turn to the writings of the twelfth-century philosopher Bernard de Chartres on the best way to learn: "A humble mind, zeal for inquiry, a quiet life, silent investigation, poverty, and a foreign land." I can follow at least some of these instructions. A humble mind, I hope; zeal for inquiry certainly; and I am seeking the wisdom of Saint Francis in a foreign land.

He is the most modern of saints, the founder of the green movement. He turned his back on materialism and property for the love of the natural world. If we are bracing ourselves for a necessary sacrifice of our resources—of energy, electricity, fashion, meat—we can look to Saint Francis as a role model. Self-denial brought him personal liberation and joy. G. K. Chesterton wrote of him: "It was not self-denial merely in the sense of self-control. It was as positive as a passion. . . . He devoured fasting as a man devours food."

Saint Francis described his epiphany from wealthy young man to friar. "When I was in my sins, just to see lepers was very bitter for me. And the Lord himself took me among them, and I showed mercy to them. And on leaving them, what had seemed bitter to me turned for me into sweetness of body and soul. And afterward I waited a little and left the world." I am captivated by that phrase: "I waited a little and left the world." He left behind the comfort of wealth to embrace the monastic principles of compassion and serving the sick. The least loved in society were most loved by him.

First, Francis sought permission from the pope to set up a fraternity, originally in an abandoned shed by a stream. The fraternity were distinctive for their hooded tunics, tied with a cord.

In *The Flowers of St. Francis*, the film directed by Roberto Rossellini, and co-written by Federico Fellini, the brotherhood assembled in rain and mud within a donkey's hovel. It was a wretched and yet beautiful tableau. It moved on to the most celebrated story in the life of Saint Francis: his preaching to the birds. This was the religious community, nature and birds. Saint Francis was indeed away with the birds. His favorites were the larks, but he dreamed of himself as a little black hen. He gave natural names to his followers—for instance, Brother Fly. He rode a donkey and picked up worms to prevent them from being trampled. Interestingly, despite this, he was not a vegetarian.

His famous prayer, Canticle of Brother Sun, praised God's creation. (I have learned that the prayer of Saint Francis of Assisi commonly attributed to him and recited with passion and some unintentional comedy by Margaret Thatcher—"Lord, make me an instrument of your peace; where there is hatred, let me sow love"—cannot be traced back further than 1912.)

From Saint Francis, there is one great lesson: the simple and profound act of communion with nature. Communion comes through a combination of wonder and empathy, and the state of mind necessary for these is humility. One of the many biographers of Francis of Assisi, Augustine Thompson, wrote: "The humiliation of the Son of God, who became a child in the stable amid squalor and domestic animals, was for Francis a model of spiritual perfection." Most of us in the secular world dread humiliation. It has become a word associated with legal rights— our self-esteem and status in the eyes of peers is measurable and valuable. For Saint Francis, voluntary self-abasement was a path to glory.

Toward the end of his life in 1225, Francis retreated to a hermit's cell. Almost totally blind, he called for the sound of a lute. His monks medicine was harsh. In an attempt to relieve the pain of his starved and exhausted body, his face was cauterized across his jaw—to no avail. What he did understand was endurance and how to die well. He returned to Assisi, dressed in sackcloth, and was sprinkled with ashes. The expression we use for extravagant penitence was real to him. On a Saturday evening just before nightfall in 1226, a flock of larks circled the cell. He died, aged forty-four, surrounded by his favorite birds.

It is July, and I am staying at a farmhouse in Tuscany, with a sloping, springy lawn, which leads down to a view of waves and waves of hillside. These are dotted with worming paths leading to hamlet churches. I can hear bells in the distance. The cobalt sky darkens to dusk blue, and the sun dips below the horizon, sending flares of pink and orange over the hilltops. This is the time when flocks of swifts swoop down to drink from the swimming pool, before thrusting back up to the sky with astonishing speed and to great heights. I am sitting on a wicker chair next to my elder son and daughter-in-law, who are expecting their first child. As the screeching air assaults keep coming, we marvel at the engineering of curved wings and forked tails; the baby kicks inside its mother's womb. We sit there until we turn to silhouettes, like the cypress and oak trees.

The following day, there is already a buzzing heat at 8:00 A.M. as I climb into the passenger seat of the rented Fiat, which my husband is driving. We are heading for Assisi on the trail of Saint Francis, whom Pope John Paul II declared in 1982 to be the Patron Saint of Ecology. I tell my husband it is about an hour's drive, although it turns out to be three. Fortunately, my husband is the patron saint of patient spouses.

Saint Francis believed that God was in Creation and therefore nature was a mirror of God. Like the old English monk, the Venerable Bede, he acknowledged time as a process of nature rather than set by man. He measured time by the sun and the moon and the seasons. His Canticle of the Creatures talks to Brother Sun, Sister Moon, wind, and water. He did not put a date on Creation, unlike the Venerable Bede—who, using the equinox, precisely dated it as March 18. But he experienced it, profoundly. Francis is pictured with a wolf at his side, which looks a bit like Evgeny's pet Boris. The difference is that Francis's wolf was tame.

He taught that nature should be a perpetual source of wonder. A collection of stories called *I Fioretta* or *Little Flowers*, written after his death, told of him stopping his companions and saying: "Wait for me while I go to preach to my sisters the birds."

I Fioretta was the inspiration for Olivier Messiaen's opera, *Saint-François d'Assise*. In one modern Paris staging of it, Saint Francis wanders across a stage filled with screen images of birds. Some critics chided the French composer for leaving out the preconversion section of Francis's life. Messiaen said: "Some people have told me: 'There is no sin in your work.' But I myself feel sin isn't interesting, dirt isn't interesting. I prefer flowers. I left out sin."

Watching birds demands an attention and patience that is at odds with the media world I inhabit. It is hard to hear anything above the babble of opinion and news feeds. But I have learned to watch and listen from a BBC correspondent named Frank Gardner, who after being shot and paralyzed by Al Qaeda while on an assignment in Saudi Arabia in 2004, remained intrepid and viscerally remembered the feel of freedom through watching birds. We once went together to the rock churches of Ethiopia, somehow managing to carry his wheelchair down vertiginous ravines. The birds that followed us delighted Frank. He photographed the blue-eared glossy starlings, the paradise flycatchers, the ceremonial-looking purple-and-green sunbird, the Ethiopian bee-eaters, with their fluffy yellow throats beneath a crest of kingfisher blue. I noticed ten birds, Frank meticulously recorded about fifty. "You just have to wait," Frank said to me. His enforced stillness liberated his mind to follow the birds. Naturally, his favorite saint is Francis of Assisi.

Other than the animals, Saint Francis's legacy is a Christlike journey toward poverty and humility. He was a merchant's son who gave away everything. A figure so close to spiritual purity that he developed stigmata.

It is also Saint Francis we have to thank for our Christmas devotion to the nativity scene. The circumstances of Christ's birth were central to him; he creatively imagined the scene and preached it. The stable, the ox, the donkey, the trough of straw. Everything we need to know is in that scene. A simple shelter, the warmth of the animals, glory in poverty and humility.

By the time we get to Assisi it is oven hot. We create a scene as we try fruitlessly to extract the parking ticket from the machine and I helpfully describe to my husband the irritation of the queue behind us. Also I am hungry, and looking for coffee and breakfast. I construct my day around appetite rather than prayer.

We walk up a steep, flagged, gray path past limestone buildings. A small group of African nuns are peering into a café, their choreography of craning heads like a ballet corps. Meanwhile, on the balconies above the street, figures are stretching, smoking, laughing. It is starting to resemble a stage set. In the square of the basilica, I spot Father Daniel Quackenbush, the Franciscan monk I have come to meet; I notice him because of his stillness rather his activity. When everyone is talking and waving, a figure who is motionless stands out.

Father Daniel is from New York and used to be a chemical engineer, but has been a Franciscan priest since 1981. He is tall, thin, bespectacled, and wears a simple Franciscan tunic and sandals. His beard is graying, his eyes kind, and his manner calm. He says that there is a private room where we can talk, but first he leads me through pink limestone arches and gleamingly worn flagstone passages to look down at the view. The Basilica di San Francesco in the old city of Assisi still worries some Franciscans. Is it too grand for a saint who preached simplicity? Father Daniel's daily pleasure is a walk through the surrounding countryside. Trees and birdsong bring him close to Saint Francis. "Birdsong can carry the spirit, sing away!"

We find a small, plain room where we can talk with a table, four chairs, and a portrait of Saint Francis on the wall. Father Daniel pours some water into a faded mug for me. All are equal here. He has shown both Angela Merkel and the king and queen of Jordan around this monastery, as pilgrims rather than heads of state. Angela Merkel was profoundly moved by the experience. Her father was a pastor who moved from West to East Germany during the Cold War because he felt needed. She experienced the spiritual potency of Assisi and wanted to learn everything she could about Saint Francis. Father Daniel also notes the connection between Saint Francis and the king of Jordan. During the Crusades, Saint Francis befriended Sultan al-Malik al Kamil of Egypt and preached respect for the Islamic faith. In 2019 Pope Francis marked the eight-hundredth anniversary of their meeting.

Saint Francis, according to Father Daniel, stood for a universal brotherhood. I ask Father Daniel how it is that Assisi still attracts five million visitors a year, many of them pilgrims. He replies that Saint Francis was authentic and the encounter feels personal. He pauses and then says there is something else. He believes that the yearning for meaning is profound and that the secular world does not lead to contentment. "People live as if God did not exist," he says. He, like G. K. Chesterton, believes that humankind must see itself in relation to the universe and time. "The earth on which we live is a spinning globe. Vast though it seems to us, it is a mere speck of matter in the greater vastness of time."

He is shocked by our ingratitude toward Creation, our carelessness toward the environment, and our distorted values. "We look for pleasure in all the wrong places," he sighs. I am interested in the religious conversion of a scientist. Surely, he must want evidence of God. Father Daniel says firmly that to him it is logical. As a chemical engineer he thought he understood how things worked, but he was always struck by a greater design. "You can look at scientific data but then think of a tiny embryo. There's design and there's design."

Since his conversion, he has found greater satisfaction working with his hands, and taken up carpentry. Science without humility, without divine love, he sees as a far greater danger than faith.

"See what happens to science when we lose our sense of the sacred—it leads to the atomic bomb," he says, agitated.

Father Daniel's brother died in a car accident, which must surely have shaken his faith. Why did God not protect him? Where is God when tragedy strikes? "Where is God? He is on the cross."

He quotes Saint Francis on the Crucifixion: "Love is not loved."

In the crypt in the lower basilica, where Saint Francis's tomb lies, the stigmata on his side, his hands and his feet are shattering to the pilgrim tourists who drop to their knees. It was not until the nineteenth century that the friars were confident that they had the body of Saint Francis. A magnificent marble tomb was built, but the brotherhood objected. Simplicity should prevail. The tomb, now restored, is made of plain pink limestone, with six candles, a cross, and simple daisies for decoration.

There is a portrait of Saint Francis of Assisi in the lower church, beneath the basilica, which is said to resemble him. He is small and thin and unassuming. By the time the Gothic painter Giotto had finished with him in his celebrated frescoes of *The Legend of Saint Francis* in the upper basilica, he was golden haired and princely. The frescoes have survived periodic earthquakes—the latest in 2016—and depict a joyous narrative of Saint Francis surrounded by nature. There are different routes to spirituality. The potency of Saint Francis owed much to the way he was interpreted in the writings of Saint Thomas Aquinas, in the poems of Dante and the painting of Giotto. Saint Francis understood the Divine Goodness that was the essence of Catholic doctrine.

Saint Thomas Aquinas wrote of the four cardinal virtues: prudence, temperance, justice, and fortitude. Saint Francis went further with his adherence to poverty, chastity, and obedience.

I wondered if the self-imposed physical harshness of Francis of Assisi were a male impulse. I imagine women in the form of Mary, nurturing rather than self-flagellating. But then I find in a pilgrim bookshop the story of Saint Clare of Assisi. Like Francis, she lived in the thirteenth century and was from a prosperous family. Inspired by Francis, she renounced everything for a life of poverty and hardship. Clare turned to the song of the sparrows, the shape of the beeches and oaks, and the feel of the wind. When she was seventeen, she ran away to the church of San Damiano, near Assisi, which became the first monastery of the Order of Saint Clare.

She took up the Rule of Saint Francis: "And observing indeed that we did not fear any poverty, labor, trial, scorn and contempt of the world, but rather that we held them as great delights, the blessed Father, moved by compassion, wrote for us a form of life." (Testament of Saint Clare). Her humility was boundless. She would kiss the feet of the sisters as she washed them. She wore a tunic of rough wool and a shirt made of boar's hair. Like Saint Francis, she used a stone for a pillow. She fasted for three days each week until Saint Francis intervened and forced her to eat a small portion of bread on those days.

There is one fresco in the Giotto series that stops you in your tracks. Blessed Francis is praying on the side of Mount La Verna, when he sees Christ crucified carried on the wings of a seraph coming down from the heavens. The six wings of the seraph might represent the six steps to enlightenment. As Francis had his vision, he felt an intense pain in his hands, feet, and side. He saw that he was bleeding. It was the stigmata. He had taken on the body of Christ.

The basilica does not feel like a tourist destination, but a place of spiritual rest. Even the groups of young visitors are quiet. Monks sit in the alcoves in poses of reflection or stroking rosaries, heads bowed. There is distant liturgical singing, which the high-ceilinged acoustics make hard to locate. Fine-looking oak pews are carved with the names of clergy.

This is the church of Saint Francis, but his spirit is surely elsewhere, at the hermitage at Eremo delle Carceri on a nearby hill, where he retreated to contemplate. The hermitage is now a pretty pink-and-white limestone priory, set within the wooded mountain. The pathway leading up to it is in leafy, dappled shade, away from the suffocating heat.

It is said to be numbingly cold up here in winter but I would be happy with its summer sanctuary. I also find, unusually, that I have lost my sense of time and of appetite; my stomach is usually a precise indicator of both. Saint Francis would have found berries and been given bread and water here. The well of Saint Francis in the hermitage courtyard is, according to legend, where Saint Francis told his followers to dig. As they did so, a spring appeared.

I have seen sacred springs before—in an Ethiopian monastery, where water rushed up at the same time each day from dry land and then stopped. Inexplicable sources of water seem both geologically natural and miraculous. Then there is the wild asparagus on this Assisi mountain, which is distinctively strong and delicious. It is enough. I realize I have bought nothing in Assisi but a postcard. It may not be great for commerce, but it is a relief. I don't need any more things.

In the centuries that followed Saint Francis's time here, various buildings were added around the hermitage, including a small friary with a little choir and refectory. Above the drystone wall near the friary entrance is an image of Saint Francis holding a circle, like a hoop. It is studded with symbols of faiths: Jewish, Buddhist, Hindu, Islamic. Saint Francis is a universal saint. His bronze face, hollowed with fasting, is lit with sunshine. He is transfigured by asceticism.

Next to that, there is another plaque with the message: Jesus Savior of Mankind. The T-shape symbol dominates. I have seen this before today in Assisi. It is the Franciscan symbol, tau, originally meaning life and resurrection. In Christianity it is an epiphany. Saint Augustine carved the tau onto people's foreheads. Saint Francis transformed himself through stigmata to a human tau—a living cross.

Around the friary, a canopy of holm oak trees forms a congregation of nature. There is one particular oak tree by the wall, which is propped up by planks. This is the tree under which the birds were said to have gathered to hear Saint Francis speak.

Looking down from the stone building, I examine the Giotto-style perspective of the land below. The wooded hills meet in a V-shaped point, and beyond this gap is a sunny expanse of land and a strip of white afternoon light. I breathe in the treetop air and the silence.

But it is also bleak. Nothing was too uncomfortable for Saint Francis. His bed was a slab of rock in a small cell. Often he would withdraw further into the woods into a cave that you could not stand up in. Its tunnel opening is today blocked by iron bars, but you can peer into the dark, dank hermit space.

There is another cast-iron statue of him sleeping on the stony ground, hard stones for a pillow, his worn feet bare. His hands are behind his head, his expression exhausted. I wish I could slip a pillow under his neck.

All is quiet, except for the birdsong. There is a gaiety to the wrens and finches at odds with the tomb-like existence of Saint Francis. Perhaps suffering made the birdsong all the sweeter. At the end of his life, foreshortened by the pain he chose, he asked a friend for cookies as his last meal. Cookies! My last meal would include spaghetti alle vongole and chocolate tart. I would want a wine list. I remembered the many-course dinners at Evgeny Lebedev's castle: the caviar and delicate fish courses, the goblets of champagne and wine. All this Saint Francis shrugged off. I walk back down the hill, with just one backward glance. A glade, a sanctuary, but also a vale of suffering.

Back in Assisi, my eye is caught by a pretty wooden door, which has the word *nun* on it. And then the word *spa*. A nunnery, which is now a luxury hotel. Society has made its choice. The impulse toward comfort is strong. I cannot understand the extreme self-denial of Saint Francis, but I have a residual sense of peace from the hermitage.

My husband and I drive back in companionable silence, at least on my side. I appreciate the smoothness of this road and the houses on the edge of it with their cheerful terra-cotta pots. Saint Francis's journeys would have been footsore, and there was no spa waiting for him.

I think about supper. We have a chef coming to the farmhouse to cook a barbecue for us tonight. I can imaginatively smell the sizzling sausages and taste the sun-ripened tomatoes and fresh basil.

That evening, I sit under a mulberry tree looking out across the Tuscan hills. My daughter-in-law is laying the table on the terrace and lighting the candles. The landscape is smudged, sky and hills blending grays and greens. I point out shapes in the clouds, convinced I can see the face of Margaret Thatcher, with her distinctive profile.

The smoke is rising from the barbecue. Soon we are clinking glasses and my appetite has returned. Family, food and drink, warm evenings, comfortable beds, and crisp white sheets. I would not want to sacrifice any of this; this is the best of living.

The following night, we drive to a hilltop restaurant for dinner in a converted monastery. The thick stone walls and plain wooden floors are simple but the restaurant is for the wealthy.

The menu is meat. Only. The first course Tuscan ham. The second an enormous blood-soaked steak, accompanied by potatoes. We gorge ourselves on the thick meaty chunks and aftertaste of fat. We clink wineglasses, smeared with the grease from our lips.

The view of the hillsides is painting-like, but there is a glinting of something else in the valley. It is the rooftops of the town, and its industrial suburbs. I can see smoke and movement of mechanical vehicles, lifting goods. While we eat like the ancient Perugians, the townspeople toil.

I sleep badly that night, my wine-soaked, throbbing mind chasing thoughts. In the morning I am out of sorts. My body cries out for cleansing. There is such a thing as excess. For the first time in my life, I decide to fast for the day. I eat one peach, dripping juice onto the ground as I walk barefoot across the grass, and after that just water or herbal tea.

By nighttime, my stomach is indignantly empty and I go to bed early. I wake before dawn, and look out of the window. A mist is rising over the blue-green hills. The birds are rehearsing. My head is as clear as a bell. The popular 5:2 diet is based on the monastic principle that fasting cleanses, body and spirit. I can at least learn from that.

Saint Francis's hardships were founded on humility rather than recovering from a hangover. But the lesson has some transference. Excess will not make us happy. We need much less than we think we do. The waste of food and clothing and the mountains of plastic landfill are testament that Saint Francis, the saint of the environment, has a legacy. We all leave the world. How will we leave the world and what kind of world will we leave?

As for birdsong, isn't it the last thing we would wish to hear before we die? After visiting the hermitage of Saint Francis, I find that I am more attuned to movements in the branches and that I can start to differentiate between garden birds. Frank Gardner taught me to notice them, but I have learned from my elderly father, a lifelong birdwatcher, how to interpret some of their songs. My father is unsteady on his feet now but his horizons are vast as he talks to the rooks on the wing in high winds.

The paradox of Saint Francis is this: His life was one of self-denial, suffering, and abasement, and yet he is a figure of joy. G. K. Chesterton again:

> *And we can say . . . that the stars, which passed above that gaunt and wasted corpse stark upon the rocky floor in all their shining cycles round the world of laboring humanity, looked down upon a happy man.*

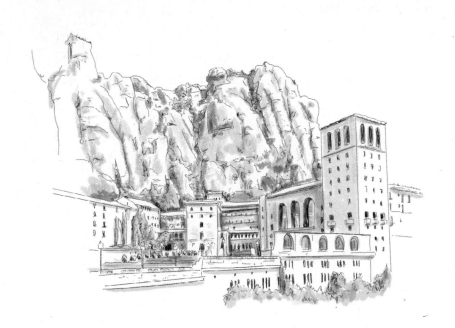

Chapter 3

THE DARK NIGHT
OF THE SOUL
MONTSERRAT, CATALONIA

O nce you become more observant of nature, you also notice the light and therefore the darkness. When I am in my office at the BBC or commuting to my nearby flat, I exist in a world of artificial light—strip lights, lamp lights, car lights. I have no sense of the gradual darkening to dusk or of the whitening dawn.

Monasteries follow Creation time rather than office time. In other words, day and night have profound meanings, rather than being overridden by work and social life. Light has a spiritual power, rising necessarily out of darkness. Think of Genesis:

And God said, "Let there be light," and there was light. God saw that the light was good and he separated the light from the darkness. God called the light "day" and the darkness he called "night."

Because monasteries are in remote places the light they inhabit is natural and the dark is unlike anything I have known in the city.

On Instagram, I follow a site about cathedrals; in the pictures, the light is draped over pillars, or it becomes a blinding revelation in windows, or performs a dramatic Caravaggio stroke illuminating darkness.

I remember a photograph of the inside of Notre Dame after the fire in 2019. It showed smouldering debris in a dimly lit nave. But the cross at the altar blazed with light. Photographers said it must have been some kind of trick of the camera lens.

Darkness and light are at the heart of monasticism. The study of Francis of Assisi led me to Saint Teresa of Avila, a sixteenth-century Spanish Carmelite nun who followed his teachings and fell afoul of the Spanish Inquisition. She, in turn, guided me to the poetry of the sixteenth-century Spanish priest Saint John of the Cross. He followed Teresa of Avila into a Carmelite order and, while staying within the sanctuary of Avila, had a vision of the crucified Christ.

He was captured and imprisoned by jealous rival orders and, in a six-foot cell, on a diet of bread and water, he composed some of his most beautiful poetry. His best-known poem is "Dark Night of the Soul." It is a term used today to express an anguished dilemma. It suggests a sort of spiritual loneliness but there is an inherent promise of morning. You cannot appreciate the light unless you have experienced the dark. Here are some verses, translated by Kieran Kavanaugh and Otilio Rodriguez, from it:

Dark Night of the Soul

1. *One dark night,*
fired with love's urgent longings

— ah, the sheer grace! —
I went out unseen,
my house being now all stilled.

2. In darkness, and secure,
by the secret ladder, disguised,
— ah, the sheer grace! —
in darkness and concealment,
my house being now all stilled.

3. On that glad night,
in secret, for no one saw me,
nor did I look at anything,
with no other light or guide
than the one that burned in my heart.

4. This guided me
more surely than the light of noon
to where he was awaiting me
— him I knew so well —
there in a place where no one appeared.

5. O guiding night!
O night more lovely than the dawn!
O night that has united
the Lover with his beloved,
transforming the beloved in her Lover.

6. Upon my flowering breast
which I kept wholly for him alone,
there he lay sleeping,

and I caressing him
there in a breeze from the fanning cedars.

7. When the breeze blew from the turret,
as I parted his hair,
it wounded my neck
with its gentle hand,
suspending all my senses.

8. *I abandoned and forgot myself,*
laying my face on my Beloved;
all things ceased; I went out from myself,
leaving my cares
forgotten among the lilies.

"Oh guiding night" is a phrase that settles. There is something about the dark that leads to understanding—a ladder in the darkness that may be hard to find but, according to Saint John of the Cross, is there to lead us out. This is the light in the enveloping darkness of the mind that most of us have experienced sometime in our lives.

Crucially, the darkness is not uniform; it has stages. The darkest part is that which comes before the dawn. It is a metaphor for hope, a promise that in the moments when life seems most bleak the sun is preparing to rise.

I have a favorite song by the Kinks, which starts: "Thank you for the days/Those endless days, those sacred days you gave me."

Two lines from it I especially love: "I bless the light/I bless the light that shines on you believe me." and "Now I'm not frightened of this world, believe me."

Saint John of the Cross wrote: "Faith, say the theologians, is a habit of the soul, certain and obscure." The more the soul is darkened, the greater the light.

In London, it is never really dark. From my flat I can see the lights of the shopping mall, the lights from landing planes, the lights from construction cranes, the dark of Grenfell Tower, the council tower block destroyed by fire and forever a tomb in the sky.

So I pack a bag on a September morning and head for the Scottish Dark Sky Observatory, near Loch Doon in East Ayrshire. You take your chances on whether it will be a clear night—and it is a risk for me embarking on a five-hour train journey. I ask the observatory if an app could not predict the night skies accurately. But they are too capricious for technology. They obey Creation time. One thing I am trying to learn in a journey toward stillness is what to try to control and what to let go.

Monasticism is an extreme form of personal discipline: The hours are exactly divided into prayer and labor. You live productively and efficiently, thought and deed controlled by a single purpose. I am trying to live more simply and tidily, since I have been to the Koyasan monasteries, and I am noticing the rhythms of nature since going to Assisi. I have bought a birdsong app to keep pace with my father. He is very old and slightly deaf, but it is I who must be armed with the latest intelligence device.

"A long-tailed tit!" I say triumphantly.

"A chaffinch," he says. "Look, it is on the top branch."

Natural wisdom takes experience and patience.

I can start by appreciating the difference between night and day. Perpetual electric daylight eclipses any chance of obtaining peace of mind. The Dark Sky Observatory removes all artificial light and reveals the depths of darkness.

I go to Scotland with my husband, my daughter, and her boyfriend; since Japan my daughter has become an Outdoor Socialist. Hiking across the country has become her alternative to politics. It beats conflict resolution, and she walks off her gloom and fears. In the pristine clear afternoon skies we walk along the wide surging river that leads to the lake. Clouds in the shape of giants pass slowly, as if being wheeled along.

We come to deep, clear, cold Loch Doon, late afternoon. The changing colors of grasses, ferns, and firs on our side are luxuriant. On the other side, the hills are craggy and bare. There is an osprey nest close by but we do not want to blunder into it, so we circle down to the pebble shore. My daughter and her boyfriend sit amid the bracken watching the sun go down. And then, with the inexplicable zest of youth, they both strip off and plunge into the icy water, their milky sculpted shapes bobbing like a mermaid and merman.

The last rays of sun dry them, and we wait for dusk to fall. Dusk is not the same as darkness. It will take another couple of hours of waiting for real nightfall.

We travel for miles looking for something to eat—village pubs offer friendly signs but keep their doors locked. The economy is darker than the skies. Eventually, we find a roadside restaurant, which makes up in quantity what it lacks in quality.

When we drive back to the national park, the darkness has no chinks. Our headlights are the only illumination for miles.

We head up an unmade road, following the headlights of the single car in front. Behind us a line of car lights forms a torch procession as the road grows steeper and bumpier. These are the Dark Skiers on their pilgrimage to witness the wonder of the heavens through powerful telescopes. On a good night, visitors can see the summer triangle, an astronomical arrangement of three of the brightest stars in their constellations.

Through a powerful telescope, we are invited to look at the rings of Saturn and the knocked-about shape of Uranus, the first planet to be identified by Herschel. We feel our way up the steps to see the space station pass brightly and cheerfully above us, like a celestial shopping cart, as close as London, orbiting the earth, seeing sixteen sunsets and sunrises a day.

There are six designated Dark Sky locations in the UK, which include Northumberland, the Brecon Beacons, and North Devon. It takes time for our eyes to adjust, and a bit longer for our spirits to accept the darkness.

Once my eyes do adjust, I feel that this is the natural order. The dark is pure calm. We drive away from the park across the moors, and in the middle of nowhere, my daughter asks if we can stop. We get out of the car, switching the lights off. There is the crowded twinkling Milky Way, there the Big Dipper, with its seven stars. The night is completely still. Silent night.

A week later I am sitting with a Church of England sister in Oxford discussing the relationship between darkness and silence. After final prayers at 8:30 P.M., the nuns enter the Big Silence, which takes them through to morning. They pray for a quiet night and a perfect end. Their final prayers are for the dead and the dying. Without wishing to belabor the significance of the dark night, it does of course bring you closer to thoughts of death. The Big Silence anticipates that silence of the grave.

The sister does not wish to be identified publicly; she regards news as an intrusion that disturbs her peaceful contemplation. Nighttime is what she waits for. She says that she avoids the *Today* program especially. Computers are used in convents, but sparingly. They are a distraction from the central gaze, the focus that comes from concentrated prayer or meditation.

I describe going to see the Dark Sky Observatory and being overwhelmed by the night skies. Nobody looked at their phones.

She nods: "The night sky, the sea, mountains, trees." It is, she says, the sense of Creation unfolding. "Out of the night, the light."

There is a place where the sky and mountains meet in a monastery that is said to be the nearest thing to heaven. This is at Montserrat, about thirty miles from Barcelona. Here, there is a sculpture by Josep Maria Subirachs called *Stairway to Understanding*. The stairway ends with a square of perfect geometry, but each step is harder than the last. The ladder of enlightenment, leading to the sky.

Montserrat is called the holy mountain; it is a fifty-million-year-old geological phenomenon, a sea gulf into which rivers poured, carrying rocks and sediment. To the eye this looks like a ridge of vertical fractures. Castles in the sky, gigantic fingers pointing at the heavens.

And here at Montserrat is a statue of the Black Madonna. The Black Madonna is a phenomenon that speaks to darkness and to light. There are many theories regarding the significance of these rare Madonnas, which are often found in trees or springs and, in the case of the Madonna of Montserrat, in a cave.

They were claimed by villagers before they were recognized by the Church and have a lineage that may date back to pre-Christian times. The Black Madonna was also Mother Earth, hence her association with caves, rivers, and trees. Her color symbolized the earth. Nuit, in Ancient Egypt, was the goddess of the night and the sky, and was sometimes portrayed as a canopy of stars spread above her husband. In Greece, Nuit became Nyx, who wore a dark veil of stars.

According to Aristophanes, Night was the beginning of creation. Before, there was only air, heaven, and earth. Night spread her black wings and placed an egg into her husband, Erebus. The egg hatched into Love, a creature with golden wings.

My husband and I arrive in Barcelona in the midst of protests over Catalan independence, and as our Ryanair flight touches down my phone pings news of a deal in Brussels between Boris Johnson and the EU. The UK is set to leave the European Union. Twitter is full of fury. All politics is upheaval.

It is a beautiful clear October day as we head for our hotel, past the industrial port and the gently rocking sailing boats in the marina. The statue of Christopher Columbus points across the seas to new lands. The horizon is shot with soft grays and pinks. The hotel receptionist says that tomorrow is a strike day, so there will be protesters in the streets and public transport will not be working. It is not a day to try to leave the city.

But I have to find a way to Montserrat. I want to see the peak that reaches toward heaven and I am entranced by the image of the Black Madonna. So the next morning we set out in search of transport. Everywhere yellow-and-red Catalan flags are draped out of windows and across the backs of students, families, the elderly. As we wander toward the center, the tarmac on the roads is jagged, where the barricades have been burning.

At the train station, there are padlocked barricades and rows of police rocking on their heels. We dart up the road to a car rental booth, aware that we need to get out of the city fast before roads start to close. We are out on the road with Google Maps just in time—as we head toward the hills, we can see the motorway bridges massing with protesters carrying Catalan flags.

The uphill road toward Montserrat has the symbol of independence spray-painted intermittently on the tarmac but I am not looking down; I am looking up. The formation of the mountains is otherworldly. The rocks look whisked up into shapes that are both beautiful and profane. As we get closer they become grander, more tumor-like, more like something from the imagination of William Blake. The skirting of larches and holm oaks prevents the landscape from looking volcanic or lunar, but it is all rather gothic.

Of the soaring peaks, one on the east thrusts higher into solitude than the rest. This is the Cavall Bernat. If you stare up, your head back, you can just about make out the statue of the Virgin on the summit.

The other peaks have more colloquial names. The Bishop, Little Chair, Elephant, Mummy. Rocks, like clouds, have anthropomorphic possibilities. I am seeing Montserrat on a clear day but it is often shrouded in mist—the monks and hermits who approached it in the tenth century must have seen it as a kingdom poised between heaven and earth.

Montserrat grew out of the monastery of Saint Cecilia, founded in the eleventh century. The mountain is still dotted with small stone hermit dwellings. The story goes that it was shepherds walking along a mountain path to the cave who discovered the figure of the Black Madonna. We follow their path.

The air is cool but with humid notes—it is somehow caressing standing here with the earth laid out beneath. In the distance, I can see the terra-cotta roofs of villages, the road, and the bridges. It's another universe. Shrubs sprout from rocks, seemingly against the odds. On the mountainside there are, according to the seasons, Pyrenean violets, honeysuckle, viburnum, and thorn trees.

This fragrant footpath is dotted with religious statues. A gaunt monk, made from seven blocks of stone, looks as if he might easily lift a carved hand in blessing. There are fifteen sculptures altogether, depicting the mysteries of the rosary: the joyful mysteries, the sorrowful mysteries, and the glorious mysteries. My husband goes a bit Anglican on all this and finds the carvings too kitsch, but I see the connection between the beauty of the surroundings and the pain and joy of the mysteries. This is a transfiguration setting.

Here, carved into the rock are the marble figures of women at the tomb of Christ, an angel seated at the edge and, above, Jesus suspended with his arms raised and golden rays surrounding his head. The resurrection of Christ carving is by Antoni Gaudí, who also designed the still-unfinished Sagrada Família cathedral in Barcelona.

Gaudí, who died in 1925, understood the potent combination of architecture, nature, and religion. He is known as God's architect. I look up from the path. The late-morning light is alabaster against the granite. The clouds are ships and funnels of steam and arcs across the sky. Continuing my little pilgrimage, I come to the crucifixion of Christ, the iron cross rising from its spiked foundations. It is on a stone platform framed by the mountain's prehistoric boulders. It is an appalling sight. The figure of Christ, held up by spikes and manacles, human suffering silhouetted against the sky.

As I climb the path to the monastery, I watch a swathe of the world descend on Montserrat. This is a place of pilgrimage. Furthermore, since someone posted on Instagram a shot of themselves on the top step of the *Stairway to Understanding*, Montserrat is near the top of the Insta bucket list.

Coaches and cars are parked half a mile down the road. If it weren't for a public strike, the railway would be bringing in more tourists. Can churches and monasteries still be described as sanctuaries? The day before I came here, I watched a young woman take a selfie in front of the table of church candles in order to show her boyfriend how flattering the light was for her. Are we able to contemplate when our attention is always on ourselves?

I have arranged to meet one of the seventy Benedictine monks here, Brother Xavier Caballé. The Benedictines are more sociable than some of the other orders, as well as being more indulgent about wine and meat. I spot him smiling at me across the square, medium height, a round boyish face, with a short graying fringe and glasses. There are no sharp edges to Xavier.

Faithful to the monk of my imagination, he produces a ring of keys from his habit and leads me through heavy doors into the monastery. All the public bustle vanishes. It is quiet and cool as we walk through the brick arches of the cloisters to the monastery garden. There is nothing left of the fifth-century monastery; in 1811 Napoleon's troops burned and sacked Montserrat.

"For no reason!" I say indignantly.

"Well, there were some troops here," says Xavier, with worldly acceptance. We walk down an arched aisle of trees along a path sprinkled with sunlight. On another path two preteenage boys in sweatshirts and jeans are strolling, the older with a protective arm around the younger. These are the boys from the Montserrat choir. The music school was set up in the fourteenth century; the oldest choir in Europe. My brother and nephew were choir boys at Canterbury and Ely Cathedral and I know how lightly these boys can wear their connection to the sublime.

I once asked a choirmaster if he could find the *Today* program a soloist for Allegri's *Miserere*, the celestial choral setting of Psalm 51. Three boys appeared. The choirmaster explained each would rehearse the soaring top C, but only one could attain perfection. One boy, one unique moment.

We reach a stone font standing in cool clear water and shaded by trees. We stop to look at the original hermitage framed by cypresses. And then Xavier beckons me to a stone bench, beneath a modern ceramic portrait of the Black Madonna, dressed in bright shades of blue, her disproportionately large hands outstretched. Baby Jesus on her lap.

Xavier, who is fifty years old, joined the Benedictines six years ago. Before that, he had a successful career as a computer scientist. He was not converted by visions, but by the welcome of another Montserrat monk. Xavier felt at home here. He says that the main difference between his present life and his old one is his constant sense of wonder: "I wake up and look out of the window, and I say, 'Wow.'"

At the end of the day he is, as storybook children might say, tired but happy. The secret of his contented existence is early rising, regimented activity, early to bed. There is a clear sense of purpose. There is little time for leisure, although he does listen to music.

"Choral music?" I ask knowingly.

"Van Morrison," he replies.

When Xavier is not attending prayers, he works in the choir school—fixing the out-of-date computers—or in the infirmary, where the older monks are cared for. The misapprehension he is keen to counter is that monasticism is an escape from life's difficulties. Imagine living in such close quarters with a community of brothers. You need to develop qualities of patience, consideration, concentration, selflessness, kindness.

Some orders have rules that politics must never be discussed, but the Benedictines permit respectful political debate. Xavier, for instance, supports independence for Catalonia. Others do not. They agree to differ. "No one owns the truth," he says. "We are only human."

Xavier has studied Saint John of the Cross and the meaning of "Dark Night of the Soul." For him, it is the story of transformation. From night to day, from darkness to light. Behind the monastery walls, life is quiet and ordered. Xavier regards the world outside now with bewilderment. "I think it is crazy," he says, with a burst of giggles. "I don't have money, I don't have a car, I don't have a house. I have what I need. I am so much richer. I can walk in the mountains, and I can think." He is studying trees and plants and wants to improve his knowledge of birdsong. It is a Saint Francis kind of existence.

He regards the material wealth of his old life as burdensome. Computers had to be upgraded, clothes updated. He worked to buy a home that he hardly saw. The release from self-perpetuating consumerism has been blissful. Can he describe his form of happiness? I ask.

"As Saint Augustine said: 'I know what time it is, but I can't explain time.'"

Xavier knows what time it is, but is too polite to mention that I am keeping him from his lunch. Before I depart, he takes me through another locked door, up and down some narrow flights of steps and into a nineteenth-century chapel of overwhelming grace and beauty.

It is decorated with mosaics and a vivid mural ceiling by the nineteenth-century Romantic artist Joan Llimona. At the center is the Madonna on her throne, welcoming the approaching pilgrims.

Xavier lifts a rope and I am a foot away from the altar, looking up at an alcove that shows the slender back of the Black Madonna, the great icon of Catalonia.

Through another door and up a few stone stairs beyond an arch of carved alabaster angels, I see the Black Madonna face-to-face. There she is, dressed in gold finery and a golden crown, seated on her silver throne. The Black Jesus on her lap. In one hand she holds up an orb—the universe—and it is this that pilgrims touch as they file past her.

Her face is long and serene, a thin straight nose, almond-shaped eyes, her lips neither smiling nor unsmiling but hovering in between. The Romanesque carving is dated to the twelfth century and a possible explanation for her color is an oxidation of varnish and centuries of candles and lamps. We cannot know for sure.

According to the academic Ella Rozett, more than thirty of the images of Black Madonnas were said to have been created by Luke the disciple. They are associated with the Benedictines, and the Cistercian monastic orders. It was the tenth-century Saint Bernard who brought the Black Madonna into Europe, through the Knights Templar. I see how she would appeal to the medieval interest in mysticism and the East. There is something Egyptian about the impassiveness of her demeanor. She could be the Egyptian goddess Isis. She is both sacred and fecund.

The dark night of the soul. The Black Madonna. I stroke the smooth orb in the hand of our Lady of Montserrat and stay a few moments longer than is fair to the queue, trying to memorize her serene expression. How could a figure signaling the birth of creation fail to have a settling effect on anxieties of the day? It is so very far away from the world of social media.

At that moment my phone pings and I surreptitiously look at it. It is a photograph of me, hand outstretched toward the Black Madonna, who is shining in her gold robes. It has been sent by Xavier, who is beaming at me. The Instagram monk.

Profoundly moved by the experience of the Black Madonna, I walk out into the courtyard and try to find my bearings. The Madonna has a concentrated power. I want to hold on to that, and I head for a museum with artistic depictions of her. The museum of Montserrat is a treasure trove of paintings by masters and modernists, including a surprisingly conventional portrait of an altar boy by Pablo Picasso.

The portraits of the Black Madonna waver between loveliness and kitsch. Here she is suspended on a cloud, the distinctive boulders of Montserrat mountain behind her.

In another, she is surrounded by angels. In a third depiction, she transcends the mountain, with the boys' choir below her. A painting by the twentieth-century artist Ramiro Fernández Saus shows her in more primitive style, with more African features, a cloud beneath her, a mountain behind.

The most contemporary depiction is a sculpture by Josep Maria Subirachs, who created the Passion Façade of the Basilica of the Sagrada Família in Barcelona and Saint Michael's Cross at Montserrat. Here, her head is a hooded shape and carved into her throne; balls are placed in formations to suggest a figure on her lap. She has the same effect in abstract: she is primordial.

The mountains, the skies, the monastery, the Black Madonna. Back in my hotel room in Barcelona that evening, I sleep deeply. What I had confronted on the visit to Montserrat was the dark night of the soul. It was the before and after, the epiphany. The Black Madonna revealed the expression of earth and sky, of day and of night.

In my secular life, I have a constant ticker tape of anxieties, some serious, some not, but all vexatious. I worry about not getting to sleep and then not waking up on time for work; I worry about logistics, travel arrangements, about professional mishaps. I worry in dreams and reality about losing my phone with all its paralyzing consequences. I worry about my children's health and happiness. Then there are the existential worries; the fears about climate and, lately, about disease. Is humankind in peril?

Monks overcome petty anxieties. They train for mastery over their thoughts and they develop a sense of equilibrium with the world through their detachment from it. I deny and fight unhappy outcomes. Monks confront and accept. Therein lies tranquility. "Behold the affairs of life," said Evagrius, the fourth-century desert monk.

Their lives are simple and ordered. They wake up on time because it is a natural rhythm. They are not overstimulated and distracted. Their lives are not ruled by iPhones. They are not disturbed by ambition and materialism. They are left with the triangle of birth, death, and faith. Their lives are not as packed as mine but they seem to be clearer and calmer. The transition from dark to light is monastic wisdom.

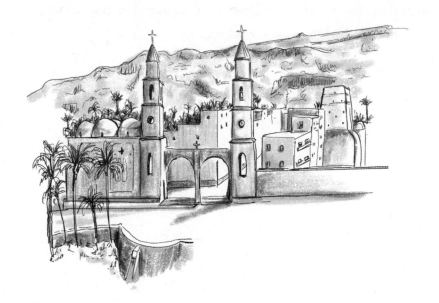

Chapter 4

SOLITUDE

THE EGYPTIAN DESERT

A utumn turns to winter, and the abbey wall at the bottom of my garden in Norfolk is laced with snow. The November sun barely rises above the wall and the barn owl disappears to hunt over a larger area of farmland. I think of the thirteenth-century nuns at prayer and labor under the tarpaulin sky.

Up until now, my observation of monastic life has been within the bounds of familiarity, an undertaking shared and socialized, in the Japanese manner. I have kept my family close. They have been living in my Hilary Mantel world for the past months, as my monastic books have started to pile up in my study.

It is time to embrace solitude, a state that is alarmingly unfamiliar to me. A writer friend once remarked to me that his perfect day was to accomplish a body of work alone in his study and then to see friends for dinner. A somewhat monastic routine. My routine by contrast is to be constantly surrounded by people from 6:00 A.M. to 7:00 P.M. and then spend time at home in the evening, catching up on emails. The antithesis of monasticism.

If I am to understand monks medicine better, I need to go back to the beginning; to the life of the desert fathers. I need to experience the merciless solitude of the desert.

A couple of years ago, I visited Cairo with the BBC's security correspondent, Frank Gardner, to watch the enthronement of the British Coptic archbishop in his ancestral land. It was a rare and elaborate ceremony in a country that was Christian long before it converted to Islam.

The disciple Mark brought Christianity to Egypt in the first century AD, and it was in Egypt that Christian monasteries first began with the desert fathers. In the fourth century the deserts of Egypt were paradoxically swarming with monks searching for solitude.

By the fourteenth century, however, Islam had become the dominant faith and the Copts are now a struggling minority, subject to continuing attacks by Islamic extremists. Frank and I traveled on a bus to the archbishop's monastery with a heavy police escort.

The year before our visit, just before Christmas 2016, a church in Cairo had been targeted, and many worshippers were killed, mostly women and children. Frank and I went to see the parents of one of those murdered in their flat, which was a shrine to the child they'd lost. The father spoke of forgiveness and martyrdom and the mother nodded agreement through suppressed heartbroken sobs. They asked Frank about turning the other cheek. After all, he had been shot and paralyzed by Al Qaeda in Saudi Arabia in 2004.

Frank replied that he had not been able to forgive, although I note that he has never spread the blame to nation or faith. Also, that he retains a verve for adventure. He is popular in these parts; the Copts have a particular admiration for his lack of vengefulness and bitterness.

The culture of martyrdom is at the heart of the Coptic religion. Perseverance and acceptance are qualities that came from the desert itself. Celebrated among Christians are twenty-one Coptic migrant laborers who were murdered by the Islamic State in Libya in 2015. Their hideous beheadings, all of them clothed in orange jumpsuits, were filmed and released as an IS recruiting tool. But it was the Copts who claimed victory, each man facing his death calmly and with prayer.

Monks are revered among the Copts, who have an ingrained memory of their suffering from persecutions. One of the most celebrated was Saint Anthony the Abbot, the "Father of all Monks," who took hold of the Western imagination thanks to his resistance to extreme temptation during his sojourn in the eastern desert. He chose suffering above pleasure, always. And he thus achieved the serenity in adversity that is the lesson of desert monasticism. Peace of mind comes through solitude and fortitude.

It is 4:00 P.M. in early November as the plane heads past Athens and the flame-orange sun is dipping beneath the horizon, with an Egyptian splendor, stretching its magenta rays like a royal procession across the sky. Why would you not have worshipped Ra, the sun deity, in ancient times? I am returning to Egypt to follow Archbishop Angaelos, whom I once watched being enthroned, back to his old monastery. He is returning to his monk's cell for spiritual renewal; I am here to listen to the silence of the desert.

I read on the plane an account of the lives of the desert fathers, introduced by Sister Benedicta Ward, based on a fourth-century record in Greek. It depicts the journey from Palestine of the first monks to settle in the desert in AD 394, and the desert truths that they revealed. The most profound confrontation with self, for a start. What the desert offers is a vast stillness.

The early Christian ascetics drew strength from the empty landscape and the burning sun. The expression they used was "freedom of heart." They found a way of living at the frontiers. Rowan Williams, the former archbishop of Canterbury, wrote a book in 2004 called *Silence and Honey Cakes: The Wisdom of the Desert*. The story of the honey cakes came from a tale about two abbots. "Two large boats floating on the river . . . in one of them sat Abba Arsenius and the Holy Spirit of God in complete silence. And in the other boat was Abba Moses with the angels of God: they were all eating honey cakes."

The lesson was that everyone is different in their understanding of spiritual life. "We live in a society," wrote Williams, "that is at once deeply individualist and deeply conformist. The desert fathers and mothers managed to be neither." As for the honey cakes, they are the food of paradise.

The most celebrated chronicler of desert monasticism was John Cassian. Born in what is now Romania, in the fourth century, he joined a monastery in Bethlehem, before traveling to Egypt, then to Constantinople. He eventually founded monasteries in Marseilles. His two treatises, *The Institutes* and *The*

Conferences, provide instructions on attaining ascetic wisdom and are still studied.

Cassian was the inspiration for the sixth-century Pope Gregory the Great, who set out to convert Anglo-Saxon Britain to Christianity, saying the Angles could be angels. The instruction is resonant: I think of the name of Archbishop Angaelos.

Saint Thomas Aquinas, the thirteenth-century Dominican theologian, also turned to Cassian for the founding principle of faith: divine revelation. The desert is a natural place to consider the soul. Jesus was tested in the desert. The Copts, who live by the principle of endurance, return there gladly.

Cassian's *Conferences* were based on his experiences in the Egyptian desert, outside Alexandria. For him, solitude—*vastissima*—was the canvas for the mind and spirit. Purity of heart was the final intention. John Cassian is still regarded as the master of the inner life.

Centuries later, in a week in November, monks have gathered to practice the same ascetic rules. Archbishop Angaelos has invited me to join him and his fellow monks and pilgrims for the trip, and sounded politely surprised when I said that I would stay the course for doctrinal discourse, but I am happy to learn about their founding saint, Saint Mark, in a place of sand and sky. The monastery, a desert community on the road from Cairo to Alexandria, is Saint Pishoy.

I meet the group at Cairo Airport. You cannot really miss the Copts in their long black gowns; sheen-black, tightly woven, circular hats; the crosses hung on chest-length chains; and their Old Testament beards. They stick together for safety, and the

Egyptian police circle them. Angaelos greets me with his combination of kindness and self-containment.

Although the Copts have a baritone look about them, they are not front of stage. They do not need an audience. Wherever they are living, they have their roots in monasticism. I have seen Archbishop Angaelos in different settings—in his Coptic residence in Stevenage, in a busy BBC studio, on television officiating at the wedding of Prince Harry and Meghan Markle. He has exuded the same calm reflectiveness in each.

As a monk at Saint Pishoy in the early 1990s, he learned the curious monastic combination of solitude within community and it has become part of his character. There is a Greek word, *nepsis*, which describes the watchful quality of monasticism in the East. Archbishop Angaelos has that quality.

After a night at the airport hotel, we continue our journey. The lobby is a mix of religious and secular—tourists heading for the pyramids navigating the pilgrims. The snatches of conversation are about God and breakfast. It is not easy herding a busload of priests, monks, nuns, theologians, and charity workers onto the coach toward Alexandria. They board quietly but not quickly. The organizer, who is also a church historian, tries to negotiate with the coach owner who wants an increased fee, before setting off. The historian, naturally, comes off worse.

Sitting in front of me is a gently spoken former monk from Worth Abbey, in Sussex; he has since been an adviser to the former archbishop of Canterbury, Rowan Williams, and to the former Labour leader Ed Miliband, so he has a combination of urbanity and innocence. He says, "I know who you are." He is referring to my job but, given the circumstances, I wonder for a second if he is staring into my soul. Nonetheless, he accepts my outsider's presence and confides his fearfulness of the committed monastic life even when he was at the gentle Benedictine monastery in Sussex. "They showed us the cells to make us penitent," he smiles. "I was terrified I would end up there."

Instead, he ended up working for the Labour Party, and then a Middle Eastern peace organization. As the former prime minister Tony Blair found, the Middle East enthralls as it frustrates. Jerusalem, the shining city on the hill, is both metaphorical and real. In medieval times, it was regarded as the center of the world, and the spiritual geography remains.

On the other side of the aisle is May, a generous, big-boned, chatty American who has come straight from Iraq and talks about it as if it were Minnesota. An easy knowledge of the Bible makes the Middle East recognizable to everyone.

We leave the Cairo suburbs with their crowded balconies of washing, plants, and A/C generators, past a vanishing glimpse of the Great Pyramid of Giza, over the flyovers, past the billboards, to the featureless desert roads. May keeps up conversation as others fall silent. She is comparing notes with Nathan, an American missionary in Albania. The conversation is jumping from doctrine to people they have encountered, to the weather.

After a couple of hours, in the unbroken pink-yellow landscape—the desert is dusty roads rather than swirling sand—we reach Saint Pishoy, in Wadi El Natrun, the most famous monastery of Alexandria. The domes and arches of its five churches rise up from the desert, surrounded by walls for both community and fortification. As the coach sways past the guards and through the entrance, the passengers, having been checked with a concentration born of experience, grow more pensive. May has stopped talking. The desert summons thought.

Inside the entrance to Saint Pishoy are some stalls selling fruit and bread, but commerce quickly gives way to prayer. Most of those on foot are monks, nuns, or pilgrims, and there is a single purpose. Here is what R. S. Thomas once described as the "hush of heaven."

The monks are accommodated either in the main building, or in cells or apartments on each side of the broom-swept, palm tree–lined central road. There are also retreats, a papal residence, and a conference building—this built in a quadrangle, its pink-brown stone and soft arches blending into the desert. What stands out is the cross, which becomes luminous at night, an answering light to the moon and the stars.

I unpack my pajamas, toothbrush, and notebooks in my single, college-style room on the second floor of the main building, before going to join the buffet lunch. The dining hall is functional and institutional but the food is pretty good and the conversation merry.

Desert monks eat lightly, once a day. In times of old their prescribed diet was bread, herbs, and water, while some monks chose to eat fruit only, or corn soup. The account in *The Lives of the Desert Fathers* describes a feast of paradise, given to the monks by angels, which included grapes, pomegranates, figs, walnuts, milk, honey, dates, and loaves. Those honey cakes again. I pile up my plate with something in between—hummus, bread, tomatoes, and cucumbers—and pour myself some water from a jug. The former monk from Worth Abbey joins me with a pilgrim, and he translates between my world and his.

I am conscious that I am a spiritual tourist here and what I really want to see are the monks' cells—the greatest expressions of asceticism and solitude. While my fellow travelers prepare for their afternoon session on the teaching of Saint Mark, I slip away. I wander up the wide, empty main street, with its avenue of trees and rows of crosses, these either on the walls or strung across the street in an arch of triumph. The crosses here are plain and victorious. There are no crucifixes, no suffering. There is none of the bustle you would expect to find in a main street, only the "hush of heaven."

Past a mud-baked wall and through an arch, I come to the main church, with its large and smaller domes, in a style characteristic of Constantinople. I wander down a narrow path to find the monks' cells. The hobbit-style proportions of the rooms come as a shock, even to someone used to London footage. Behind the low wooden doors, there is only enough space to accommodate a mattress. Each door is marked by a cross.

Larger rooms are available—of the type that Archbishop Angaelos inhabited when he was a desert monk—but some monks still prefer the original cells. The greater the ascetic discipline, the purer the self, they believe. If you close the exterior, the interior works harder, like a muscle. To me, the cells look like tombs rather than rooms, but I remember the advice of the medieval abbots, that life is best led as an antechamber to death.

The old monastery itself is simply laid out—a refectory, an ancient garden, a mill, a library, the cells, and in the courtyard, a well, known as the Well of Martyrs—due to the gruesome legend that after a massacre of forty-nine monks at the monastery by marauding Berbers, they washed their swords in the well's water.

Next to the monastery enclosure is the paradoxically grand and simple Copt cathedral, with its distinctive arches and curves and the cross on the dome.

All is quiet at the monastery as I walk around it alone in the gentler heat of the afternoon. Some monks are strolling, stopping to bless passers-by with their chains and crosses. At the edges are ever-watchful security guards. I recall the enthronement of Archbishop Angaelos here, a couple of years ago, when Frank Gardner, the producer Jonathan Harvey, and I watched the liturgy and blessing—we started to wilt after the first three hours. Copts do not cut these things short. Indeed, they boast that a normal service allows about forty-one refrains of "Kyrie Eleison."

When the service was finally over—you could never be quite sure—we stretched our legs in the pleasant courtyard garden and wondered at the harmony of the community. A production team can get tired and scratchy on just a week-long assignment. How was it living in close quarters with a brotherhood, all your life?

On that visit, we traveled to a second monastery nearby named Saint Macarius, a place of remarkable peacefulness, surrounded by pink- and orange-flowered bushes. On the hillside lived hermits, in mud brick houses; people would leave their food outside for them. It seemed a kind of oasis. One of the monks led me around the gardens, where they grew mint and thyme, and fields of crops.

I asked him, "How did the first desert monks live? There was no life in the desert, not a plant, nothing." He replied, "If you need sustenance, you find it." He stopped in an orchard to pick a branch of orange blossom for me. I smelled it, piercingly fresh and lovely. The monk and I had nothing in common except for our shared love of this fragrance. I can still see in my mind the monk holding out the white flowers, an egret on the ground behind him, still as stone. Whenever I smell orange blossoms, I think of him.

About a year after our visit for the enthronement, as I was fixed at my computer in the BBC office in London, I saw out of the corner of my eye Frank Gardner wheeling himself at speed toward me. He was bringing news of the violent death of the abbot, Bishop Epiphanius, at the monastery of Saint Macarius.

The abbot had been struck across the head as he made his way to attend Midnight Praise. At first the police thought they were investigating terrorism, but the killer had to have known the daily rituals in order to know when to strike. Two monks from Saint Macarius were eventually found guilty. Their grievance was theological.

The Coptic Pope Tawadros II pleaded, "Stand firm . . . our monasteries are fine. Monasticism will triumph."

◦ ◦ ◦

I return from my walk around the monks' cells to find the afternoon session is underway. The room slightly resembles a funeral parlor with its flower arrangements and box of tissues on the center table. But the meeting itself is more like a council. A square-shaped table, microphones, notebooks, water bottles. What makes it otherworldly is the central figure of the patriarch, His Holiness Pope Tawadros II.

He is of immense height, with large features and a long white-gray beard. With his hands clasped over his scepter, he looks like Sarastro, the priest from *The Magic Flute*. Mozart's opera was imagined in Egypt. The head of the priesthood, Sarastro, representing light and reason, must ward off the revenge of the Queen of the Night, who represents passion and chaos. My daughter describes it as patriarchal propaganda.

Yet, here is Pope Tawadros welcoming a woman academic to read out her paper on Saint Mark. He is the saint of the Egyptian desert—he came from Libya to set up the first desert monasteries in Egypt, and blessed Saint Anthony, becoming the first pope of the Coptic Orthodox Church.

In his deliberate, rumbling, patient manner, Pope Tawadros then describes the monastic way—mercy, joy, study, prayer. Archbishop Angaelos adds a reminder of the Coptic monastic creed. Tolerance is not enough. Copts are bound to love their enemies.

Very different in temperament, the next speaker is the Anglican bishop of Egypt, named Mouneer Anis, just arrived from Alexandria. A fleshy, good-humored-looking man who is a physician and a painter as well as a bishop, he nevertheless shakes his head over what he describes as the "joy, joy, joy, dance, dance, dance, jump, jump, jump" offer of the evangelicals. Churches, he says, should not be sites of entertainment.

Looking around the room, he tells us that we should recognize that joy and suffering are twin states in life and you must never deny the suffering. The monastic life of hardship is a perpetual reminder that this is so.

Monastic truths give you an appetite and I am grateful that this is not a fasting day. Back in the functional dining room, I pile my plate up with bread, hummus, herbs, chicken, and salad. It was fourth-century Egyptian monasticism that formed the basis for Egyptian cuisine and health. Dried bread, green herbs, olive oil, beans, and lentils are all monastic fare. The wheat the monks grew, meanwhile, was sent off to Alexandria, known as the port of hedonism. *Historia Monochorum*, a text about monasticism in the fourth century, claims that the monks could make the desert blossom. Plants and herbs that had never been seen before flourished.

As for the tradition of two days of fasting—Wednesday and Friday—this has become the foundation of the 5:2 diet, the world's most successful diet. "Eat less" is monastic in its simplicity.

As I tuck in, a tentative figure approaches my table. His plate is only half full. It turns out that he is a Syrian Christian and a professor at the University of Salzburg. His dream is to save his culture from being erased. If he could just bring manuscripts from the diaspora to Salzburg he could recreate Alexandria—a university and a monastery in the manner of Saint Mark. He sees monasticism as the spread of civilization. By the time our plates are empty, we are getting on famously, and agree that I must visit him in Salzburg, and help him fight for his library.

But now it is time for the evening doctrinal session. The bowed heads contemplate the role of Saint Mark, who wrote the first of the four Gospels and brought Christianity to Alexandria, where he was captured and dragged through the streets with a rope around his neck until he was dead.

The name Alexandria is on the lips of all here—as a frontier of civilization and of faith.

In a Dan Brown–style twist, I learn that more than twenty other Gospels were destroyed following the fourth-century Nicaea summits on the nature of the Holy Trinity, but fragments of Saint Mark's Gospel and Judas's Gospel survive in a village outside Cairo.

Meanwhile, Saint Mark's relics are said to be kept in a shrine in the Coptic church of Alexandria, although some were taken to Venice. "You should go," says my sad, smiling Syrian friend. "You will love Alexandria." As I walk back to my room, I have a message from the British ambassador in Cairo, who has heard that I am here, and is curious about my mission. He invites me to dinner and advises me first to get to Alexandria if I can. Again. All roads, at least from here, lead to Alexandria.

My room card is blank, but I think I remember the number. Unfortunately, I do not, and as I try various doors, blameless worshippers open them, puzzled and anxious to help. There is quite a crowd by the time I find my room, so I gratefully shut the door and am at last alone. It is like a smaller version of a Travelodge room. There is space for a bed, a table and a wardrobe, and no more. The confinement is oddly liberating.

I open the window and breathe in the dry desert air. My thoughts are lucid. The desert monks were said to have had extraordinary dreams of angels, and they found that they could prophesy. *The Lives of the Desert Fathers* cites "nature miracles." The monk Bes was said to have been able to commune with animals—in the manner of Saint Francis. He even made friends with the crocodiles. Indeed, one fellow desert monk used a crocodile as a ferry across the Nile. The Egyptian desert made visionaries of the truly humble. The greater theme was that desert monks were restored to the time before original sin; the desert became a kind of Garden of Eden.

In the desert evening, I feel at peace. I am in a monastic settlement; I have a plain, clean room and windows that look out to the vastissima of desert and sky. The community has become an oasis of light. The whole place is lit up by lanterns and the cross at the top of the dome is radiant.

John of Lycopolis, the desert hermit, instructed: Cultivate stillness and train yourself for contemplation. In the desert, this cannot be faked. Those seeking monastic virtue are warned of the distinction between wanting to seem good and being good. John talked of the "serpent wrapped round the heart." The restless heart fights against inner peace and stability, which come from the virtues of the desert: love, meekness, sufferance, not judging. I think I glimpse what is meant by the "huge silence" of the desert. It is my own invisibility within the grand scheme of Creation. I want to cast myself into the desert air.

I wander about shutting the curtains, but the night is so beautiful that I keep the window wide open and the soft, cold air fans me to sleep. My head is on the flat pillow, my mind is among the stars.

I am woken by the high-pitched whistle of a mosquito around my head, and then count a couple of others coming from different directions. I try to hide under the single sheet and the almost rock-hard pillow. But I need to breathe, so surface for air and find the angry buzzing waiting for me.

I go to shut the window but it is too late. The enemy is within. Round and round my head in a vicious ring-around-the-rosy. This continues well past midnight. I fetch my skirt from the wardrobe and wrap it around my head to form a kind of burka. Only my nose and part of my cheeks are exposed; I beg for mercy. At about 3:00 A.M. I give up and open the window again. Perhaps the mosquitoes will tire of me. I am furious and self-pitying. Why did I ever open the window in the first place? I scowl at the cross outside, fading slightly as the night passes from blackness toward the dawn.

As the birds begin their matins—oh, at last the dark night is over—I pull my throttling skirt from my head and go to the basin to wash my face. I catch a glance of myself in the mirror. I look as if I have some kind of medieval pox. My nose is livid red, and on closer look my face is a mountain range of bumps and blisters. My cheeks have spots like felt-pen dots across them. Now I know what is meant by the expression "eaten alive." I must have dozed and my face covering slipped.

I should be forbearing, but I am mortified. I am leaving to go to the fabulous, cosmopolitan city of Alexandria, in the footsteps of Saint Mark. And then I am returning to Cairo to dine with the British ambassador and his wife. And my face is now a scarlet crater.

I paint on some Elizabeth I–style thick strokes of foundation, stick on some dark glasses, in the manner of postcosmetic surgery and, mustering what dignity I can, head toward the entrance to the monastery. I pull at several bolted wooden doors until I find a little open gate in the wall, and slip through. As I look back, the Church historian who has organized this trip is viewing me quizzically, hands on hips. Fortunately, it is a first principle of the Coptics not to judge.

I wait at the entrance for the taxi. The stall holders are setting up, quietly and purposefully, as if preparing Communion. I try to hide my face from them, a vain and embarrassed woman.

While I am waiting, I take from my rucksack a book. It is called *Harlots of the Desert*—a study of repentance in early monastic sources, translated by Benedicta Ward.

She writes of a Mary Magdalene, called Mary of Egypt. A female saint, known in the sixth century, her story is one of penitence and redemption. She lived a dissolute life in Alexandria until she joined some pilgrims traveling to Jerusalem. At the door to the Church of the Holy Sepulchre, she wept with contrition. The next day she crossed into Jordan and lived in the desert for forty-seven years as a hermit in penitence. The lesson of Mary of Egypt is that the most lustful and wicked woman or man can be redeemed. Virginity is Christ-like. Lust becomes love. Vanity worthless. There is hope for all of us.

The great purpose of desert monasticism is to master self-consciousness, appetite, and passion. John of Lycopolis promised that true desert monasticism would bring an end to anxiety. The less you have, the less niggling your desires and worries.

Alas, that I leave the place more concerned by the insect bites on my swelling nose.

But on the desert road, my fretfulness begins to pass and I doze off. When I wake, the roadside has changed. Amid the sands and the scrubs, I spy cranes poking about for food. And then verdant grass that turns into green islands among glinting water. We are approaching the vast port of Alexandria.

Ports represent trade and movement of people, conquerors and conquered. Alexandria was founded in 332 BC by Alexander the Great, one of the greatest of conquerors. But its glamor is peeling and faded. The city still has the aspect of a gateway, but cries out for the bustling trade of ancient times.

One of the recent peace proposals for the Middle East had the imaginative vision of opening up Gaza, making Egypt and the Suez Canal busier and recreating Alexandria as the portal to the Mediterranean and Europe. Walking around here, you can easily imagine this. The ancient city of Alexandria is buried, but you know that it is there, under the hotels and apartment blocks. And the people here have a knowing air about them. I have seen it in Lebanon's Beirut, another port. There is an ease, an exhilarating openness, a sophistication. Many are young. Some women cover their heads, others do not. They sit in groups on the harbor wall, talking intently, but also laughing.

I look round a Roman excavation site and wonder at the size of the public baths, and indeed the weight of the marble on display. This was a place of learning and pleasure. It was here that Antony fell in love with Cleopatra. The Alexandrians claim to have found her burial site and will one day excavate the watery tomb.

At the end of a peninsula is the site of the lighthouse of Alexandria, now a fortress. The lighthouse, over three hundred feet (one hundred meters) high, was a wonder of the ancient world, like the Colossus of Rhodes. Nothing like it had been seen before, a beacon to the seas, a magnet for the Middle East. I look out at the flotilla of bobbing boats in the harbor and the

Mediterranean expanse beyond—the West one way, the East in the other.

I remember the lines spoken by Enobarbus in Shakespeare's *Antony and Cleopatra*:

The barge she sat in, like a burnished throne,
Burned on the water: the poop was beaten gold;
Purple the sails, and so perfumed that
The winds were lovesick with them; the oars were silver,
Which to the tune of flutes kept stroke, and made
The water which they beat to follow faster,
As amorous of their strokes.

I can picture the shape of this barge, coming into the harbor of Alexandria. This is where both temptation and martyrdom arrived—from Libya, from Jerusalem, and from the Mediterranean. In 385 Jerome arrived in Alexandria after traveling through Palestine from Syria. During the same period John Cassian arrived from a monastery in Bethlehem.

The civilization here was magnificent—a contrast to the frugality of the desert. The great library of Alexandria, built in 285 BC, was one of the largest libraries in the world and made the city famed for its learning. A new modern library, dominating the old city, houses old artifacts and modern works. It is full of students and professors, heads down, reverent.

The library feels part museum, part concert hall in its enlightened self-respect. I think of my Syrian Christian lunch companion at the monastery and his ambition to recreate his civilization. My eyes fill with tears at the thought of his love for his country, devastated by war.

To complete my monastic journey here, though, I must leave the harbor and head into the old city to find the relics of Saint Mark. These are kept in Saint Mark's Coptic Cathedral, a heavily guarded church in a maze of streets. A guard asks me for my passport, and I tell him that I am so sorry but I have left it in the car. He looks at me, both belligerent and fearful.

He asks, "Christian?" I nod. He looks torn, but jerks his head toward the entrance. I can go in. His suspicion is based on some experience. A couple of years ago, an IS sympathizer detonated a suicide belt in this cathedral, killing seventeen people.

I walk silently, and almost alone, up the central aisle, past the wooden pews. I look up at the images of the disciples. There is Saint Mark, who came here two thousand years ago. A church warden takes me to a closed room at the side, and I look at a glass cabinet, in which richly colored and decorated rolled cloths are laid on shelves. These are said to be the relics of Saint Mark.

I turn to smile at the church warden and he looks back kindly at my pox face, as if I have come to the relics hoping for a cure. There is a picture of Saint Mark in a smaller church that is easier for me to grasp. Here he is, landing in Alexandria, a lion at his feet. There is a ship in the water, and the lighthouse of Alexandria is visible. In the distance are the pyramids. Saint Mark, the founder of Christianity in Africa, has landed in Egypt.

On the road back to Cairo, I am flooded with thoughts about the desert fathers. They came in search of suffering, in order to experience joy. For monks such as Saint Anthony, it was a profound test of faith and character. Would solitude and hunger make one more vulnerable to temptation? Saint Mark tested himself, following the temptation of Christ in the Judaean desert. We all need to question our moral resilience.

I try to make sense of my desert experience. My night of sleeplessness was in fact quite monastic. An Egyptian saint named John the Hermit prepared for his life as an ascetic by standing under a rock for three years. "One night's sleep is enough for a monk if he is a fighter," as one monastic saying goes.

As the sun sets over the River Nile, I reach Cairo. Sunbaked, pox-faced, and dirt-streaked, I enter the gates to the manicured lawns of the British embassy. The ambassador and his wife are on the steps of the white mansion to greet me. They are too diplomatic to mention my appearance, and I suddenly do not care what I look like. What would Bishop Angaelos do? He would be a monk, whatever his circumstances. I raise a toast to monasticism and I think of nepsis. Be still.

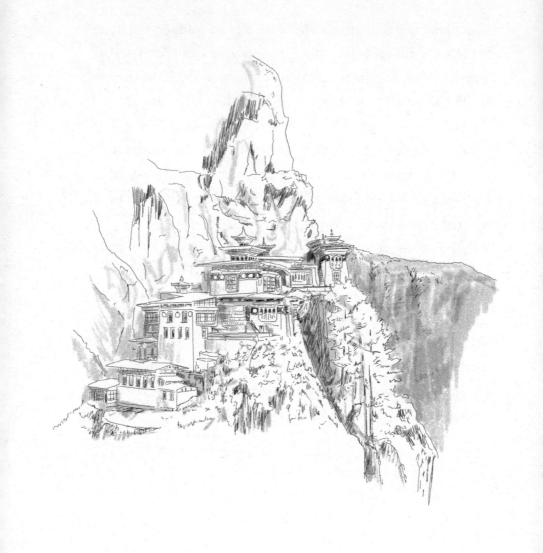

Chapter 5

THE ART OF HAPPINESS AND SAVING THE PLANET
BHUTAN

I n the Egyptian desert, monks did not talk of happiness, but of humility and purity, experienced in the huge silence. Eastern monasticism has a different expression. It is Abiding Calm. This is at the heart of happiness.

The small Himalayan country of Bhutan has made happiness its purpose, so it seems the best place to seek it.

Britain, like many other countries, likes to talk about its national identity. It happens every year, for instance, at the BBC Proms, a series of classical concerts at the Royal Albert Hall ending with an exuberant last night—"Rule Britannia," sea shanties, flag waving. Some people get cross, saying that this is a jingoistic celebration of Empire and colonial rule. Others say, what are we but a seafaring nation with a queen?

America might say that its founding principles are God and freedom. France has liberty, equality, and fraternity. China's state is built on Mao, most appealingly his maxim of "letting a hundred flowers bloom."

Bhutan has decided that it stands for happiness and has constructed its economy around this abstract. In 1972, it replaced the conventional economic index with its own Gross National Happiness Index. The index measures the country not just by economic growth but by criteria such as health, education, and "psychological well-being."

Economists such as Richard Layard have tried to introduce the happiness index to the UK, calling for governments to assess the impact of their policies on personal happiness. One of the striking decisions made by Bhutan was to put climate above economic growth. This landlocked country, located in the eastern Himalayas, is carbon negative. It has a population of less than a million and it is strict on its visa admission to visitors from other countries. It deliberately limits its tourism. In a way, it anticipates the kind of society that others might turn to in the future. Controlled borders, public health first, community before nation.

Bhutan has built its society on a monastic code of simplicity. It practices the same kind of Buddhism as Tibet, which lies to the north. It is not happy out of naivety. Bhutan knows how geopolitics works and keeps a wary eye on the neighboring superpowers of India and China. Happiness is a choice—of politics, temperament, lifestyle, and faith.

So in search of big smiles I board the plane for Thailand with my husband at Heathrow, on the first leg of our journey to Bhutan. There are no direct flights; Bhutan's airport is about the same size as that of a provincial town.

I put my passport in the seat pocket, fasten my seatbelt—and sit back and think of lichen.

The first sign of a healthy environment is the appearance of lichen, and on the wooded slopes of Bhutan there is an abundance of it, which serves as a metaphor for its society and for my peace of mind.

I am leaving behind a scene that deeply lacks lichen. Britain is in the maelstrom of an election campaign; the media have fallen out with the politicians and Twitter is at its most trigger-happy. At work we are surviving on coffee, cold pizza, and hyper news. Instead of abiding calm, there is sound and fury.

The book that I read on the flight to Thailand is *The Tibetan Book of Living and Dying* by Sogyal Rinpoche, a Tibetan lama. He writes:

> *Modern society seems to me a celebration of all the things that lead away from the truth, make truth hard to live for and discourage people from even believing that it exists.... The modern samsara feeds off an anxiety and depression that it fosters and trains us all in, and carefully nurtures, with a consumer machine that needs to keep us greedy to keep going.... The key to finding a happy balance in modern lives is simplicity. In Buddhism this is what is meant by discipline. Peace of mind will come from this. You will have more time to pursue the things of the spirit and the knowledge that only spiritual truth can bring, which can help you face death.*

All that matters is love and knowledge.

We stop for the night in Thailand before the flight early the following morning, glad of a fancy hotel, cocktails, a profusion of towels. It takes effort to be weaned from comfort and glamor.

Thailand is an economic powerhouse, and in forging its way it has sacrificed some of the innocence of Bhutan. A giant billboard near the airport calls for respect and dignity to be shown toward the image of Buddha. It warns that it should not be used in bars, or on tattoos.

Another government advertisement begs the population to cut down on their iPhone consumption to save electricity. On a boat ride up the Chao Phraya River, we pass the old palace and a new one—Siam Icon, a dazzlingly lit luxury shopping mall, Gucci emblazoned across the night sky. I fondly remember the luminous crosses on church domes in the Egyptian desert.

Bhutan, until recently thought quaint, could be ahead of us all. A Singapore minister once gave a speech about its own growth economy, comparing it to the "backwardness" of Bhutan. A Bhutanese journalist wrote in reply: "It would take Bhutan ten years to be like Singapore. Who knows the length of time it would take for Singapore to get to be Bhutan."

Seventy percent of the country is forest. Its symbols are the Himalayan cypress and the national flower—the Himalayan blue poppy. I look at pictures of this flower, which looks like something out of a fairy tale with its vibrant blue petals. But somehow seclusion and faith make anything possible. Bhutan offers an alternative model to globalization—peaceful self-sufficiency and monasticism over materialism.

Queuing at Bangkok airport, we watch a twenty-two-inch Samsung television being loaded on with the luggage in front of us. The design of airports—and shopping malls—caters to a different kind of satisfaction than the happiness of Bhutan. The malls are sterile, without season or weather. A lengthy wait here gives me plenty of time to shop and lower my spirits.

It is a relief to board the Bhutan Airlines plane at sunrise and watch the impressionist dabs of pinks and grays and a sheep-shaped, wavy, soft gray cloud, which I consider posting to the Cloud Appreciation Society. My attention to clouds since writing this book has been serotonin-enhancing. The national colors of Bhutan—yellow for state, orange for monastic authority—daubed across the plane are in the same spirit of cheerfulness.

We fly over Indian plains and peaks, not sure what is low cloud and what is snow. It is December, but snow-capped mountains are a less common sight because of climate change. In the northwest are the peaks of Bhutan: the only mountains in the Himalayan range that cannot be climbed.

During the second half of the twentieth century, Bhutan effectively nationalized happiness, defying many of the world's global conventions. It was the third king, Jigme Dorji Wangchuck, who believed that the sacred trumped human demand and desires; he turned happiness into a political project. Deciding that the chasm of social inequality made people unhappy, he dictated that nobody could own more than twenty-five acres and everyone would be given five acres to make a start.

But happiness is fragile and so is Bhutan. It fears contagion from the outside world. There are strict laws on foreign ownership—which can only happen when a majority share is owned by native Bhutanese. Tariffs are imposed on all visitors—warm hospitality combined with taxes. India, as one of its closest neighbors, has been exempt, but this policy is now being reconsidered. The aspiration of Bhutan is to give preference on jobs to its own people, but even Bhutan cannot do without migrant workers. Fifty thousand out of a population of eight hundred thousand are foreign, mostly Indian. Bhutan keeps an eye on numbers—letting in enough migrants for the economy, without risking affecting the culture.

Bhutanese history has a mythological cast. The country is said to have been created by a saint and a Buddha named Guru Rinpoche, who came from Pakistan, flying on the back of a tiger to suppress demons in the mountains. For the rest of us, planes are easier.

The fierce purity of high-altitude air hits me as we come down the plane steps and we drink in the scene of mountains and rivers. The airport building is traditional, white walls and decorated wood, no statement modern architecture here.

Waiting at Arrivals, about as busy as a bus queue, is Tenzin Phuntsho, who chose to be a guide rather than a monk but who nevertheless retains his monastic composure. He has a wide, curious face and military-short black hair, and he wears the Bhutan costume of a checked knee-length gown with woolen tights. He hands us a glass bottle of water and an apple from a local orchard. There is a ban on most plastics in Bhutan.

Tenzin says winter food in west Bhutan is limited, although improving roads allow vegetables to come from the south. He does not even raise the idea of importing food; it is a simple assumption that food should be familiar and seasonal.

Later we stop for a lunch of cabbage, oyster mushrooms, chilies, red rice—a staple here—and cheese. There are no gastro restaurants, just small rooms at the top of linoleum staircases—and we phone ahead to order. The food is cooked for us, and nothing is wasted. I look out of the window at the mules and oxen and ploughs among the bicycles. Bhutan has the rural simplicity of other Himalayan countries I have visited—such as Ladakh in the region of Kashmir. But there is also scholarship here and a culture of chivalry, thanks to the monasteries. The young royal family are friends of William and Kate, Duke and Duchess of Cambridge.

We stroll along the glacier river. It is a pure greenish hue and transparent; beneath it, the large stones and pebbles appear like glistening glass shoes. Above us is the Ringpung Dzong, the seventeenth-century "fortress of heaped jewels" that houses not only the district monastic body but also the government offices. The state is literally and metaphorically created out of monasticism.

It is also part of everyday life. There is a gesture performed in prayer before Buddha thrones, which are plentiful in Bhutan. You put your palms together and gesture to your forehead, mouth, and chest. It brings together mind, speech, and heart. It is a rebalancing of the fallen state represented by the three poisons of ignorance, anger, and greed.

The Buddhism of Bhutan warns against dislocation—from nature and from others. Monks who study during their three years of meditation do so within a natural landscape in order to absorb the truths of mountains, trees, rocks, wind, rivers. Before Buddhism was introduced to Bhutan in the seventh century, its religion was animism—the Bon religion. Buddhism did not try to eradicate the Bon religion; it merged with it.

Nature is part of monks medicine. I watch a house being blessed by a monk swinging incense around the newly completed upper rooms. All houses here are built to the same pagoda-like design, in accordance with the Bhutan style—conformity of style leads to aesthetic serenity. The incense used by monks contains herbs and plants from the mountain—juniper and cypress are meant to be especially healing.

The other philosophical principle of Bhutanese Buddhism is turning a negative into a positive. Guru Rinpoche came to Bhutan to subdue the bad spirits. This is a continuing mission. Tenzin wears an amulet around his neck. People here are good by design and will—they are always aware of lurking sins.

The festivals of Bhutan are based on ritual ceremonies of triumphing over bad spirits. The monks who perform these masked ceremonies prepare by meditating themselves into a state of enlightenment so that goodness enfolds the audience. In Bhutan, virtue is not private but societal and inherited.

Bhutan looks for symmetry and harmony. This is even demonstrated in the current monarchy—the former king has abdicated but lives in Thimpu near his son, who is in his forties, now reigning and raising his own son. "Past, present, future," says Tenzin contentedly.

A room at the little museum in Paro is dedicated to pictures of flowers and wildlife. The blue poppy, the little rose finch bird, the swallowtail butterfly, the rare snow leopard. We walk back down the path in the warmth of the sun, the shocking purity of the air, the hills covered in cypress, maple, pine, and fluttering prayer flags.

We follow the river road toward Thimpu, which is regarded as a big city—certainly a center of population. We pass yellow, green, and red prayer flags fluttering from wire lines, and houses of whitewashed walls and wooden roofs in the distinctive Dzong fortress style. Even the king's palace in Thimpu follows the style—pretty rather than splendid. The only outsize monument is the imperial one-hundred-sixty-five-foot- (fifty-meter-) high bronze Buddha looking down from the mountain, donated by the Chinese with the express purpose of bestowing peace and blessings on the whole world.

We book into an almost empty hotel, with the dining facilities of a 1950s English seaside boarding house. It is fair to say that Soho House has passed Bhutan by. A short burst of Wi-Fi at reception flashes the repercussions of a terrorist attack on Westminster Bridge, London, the standoff between the BBC and the Conservative Party over the lack of access to Boris Johnson, and remarks by the retiring BBC anchor David Dimbleby that the election is vile and that social media has destroyed civility. I shudder.

The temperature drops at nightfall, so we wrap up and find a nearby restaurant tucked behind an anonymous entrance. We settle down to yak stew (similar to oxtail) and dahl. The wine is like paint stripper, and I remember to order beer next time. Outside, it is Saturday night in the city but the only sound to be heard is a musician on a lute and some accompanying foot tapping.

We strike up a conversation with an entrepreneur who talks of reconciling ambition with happiness. "The internet means comparing lives with people whom we do not know, which introduces both possibility and discontent."

Our companion earns enough to send his daughter to a boarding school over the border in India. It makes his wife sad and his daughter homesick and increasingly detached. His dream is to get his daughter into Cambridge. So far, so Western.

His other concerns sound less Western. He does not want his striving to lessen his sense of blessings. He talks of balance, of community. For instance, before someone builds a house in Bhutan they must ask permission of those around them, rather than just going through a legal process. No desire can be seen in isolation of its effect on others.

During mountain treks, guides pay ceremonial respect to the nature of each district as they enter and leave it. Buddhist monks teach that we are stewards of the land and must leave it as we find it. A sense of harmony is priceless.

Our dinner companion says that national harmony is preserved by the belief that his country has control over its destiny. The population decided that it did not like traffic lights, so the country does without them. Everyone who chops down a tree has to plant two in its place. Each June, they celebrate Environment Day by planting trees in school grounds. Students then take responsibility for the care of the trees they have planted. This is how the government of Bhutan prescribes peace of mind.

At the heart of everything in Bhutan is the monastic mission. It is the monks that I must join.

After a chilly, sweaters-and-bedsocks night in our guesthouse and a breakfast of boiled eggs, we head for the mountain monastery. We clamber into a small minibus, which creeps up the mountain path, navigating stones, tree trunks, and the occasional vehicle coming the other way on a single track, so we have to pull precipitously over to the edge.

Then the minibus stops in an opening at the start of the wood and we begin our ascent on foot.

It is a hot-and-cold day in winter sunshine. I pull off layers of sweaters then put them back on when the sun goes into the clouds. The sky is blue behind the blue pines and oaks of the mountain forest.

We carry an overnight bag for the monastery. I am guessing that it will be freezing, and I don't expect to get undressed. The pine needle–covered path is steep and winding. I stop to take a breath, kicking a stone, which bounces down into the valley. I look down at the broad glacier river, the expanding town shrinking with perspective.

Thimpu is really a model settlement surrounded by forest mountains. I can see the rooftops of the royal palace and the government offices. The palace looks modest and feminine from this angle. You must be able to hear the river from the bedrooms. Up along the sandy forest path, I am inhaling the smell of pine and lichen-clean air as if it is incense. And as I steadily ascend, my thoughts become clearer too. At the base, they are the usual circular collection of lists and reconstructions. It is a social media mind, looking for the next thing, full of judgment and irritability. As the altitude increases, and the sun grows hotter where we cross its spotlight, my mind starts to quieten. Priorities take shape—sorrowful thoughts about the victims of the terror attack, solicitous thoughts about my pregnant daughter-in-law.

I remember the pictures of Buddhist progress, which look a bit like this mountain path. At the lower path, there are distracting monkeys at your back. As you get higher, you start to conquer some of the demons. Your mind and spirit begin their purification. I take deep breaths of alpine air, which do not require thought.

Further up the path, reaching the summit of the hill, the bracken is brown for winter and the trees are skeletal. Here is a decorated wooden hut, with carved patterns beneath its roof. And there are some figures walking down the path—they go from specks to a round-faced boy of about ten years old, in yellow robes, hand in hand with a monk in claret robes. The boy has a preternatural confidence. I realize that he is leading the monk rather than the other way round. The boy is holding a silver-topped stick and has a spring in his step. He greets me cheerily.

The guide whispers that he is a child lama—a reincarnated boy with special powers. Lamas are spotted through unusual early behavior. This often includes a detailed interest in a place they have never seen. Another monk behind the boy stops for a chat. Where are we from? He is from Ladakh, the land I had visited in northern India, close to Tibet. Another place of monasteries in the Himalayan mountains, with rivers, yaks, pastures; another small haven eyed up by the superpowers of India and China.

A little further and we walk into a clearing. There are goalposts at either end of it. I comprehend the strangeness of this. It is a football pitch at the top of a mountain. It turns out that the abbot is much more liberal than his peers and is fond of football. He cajoles all the young monks into engaging in tournaments in between prayers. The path has started to wind down now, clouds eclipsing the sun. The weather is changing; cold mist descends fast on the mountain.

Nailed to the trees are encouraging messages for visitors and pilgrims, written in yellow on red-painted wood. The first says: "No road is long with good company." The view down from the path is nothing but firs, and a shaft of sun laser-lights its own heavenly path.

My husband walks ahead with the heavy pack, which I joke to Tenzin includes a bath, a Deliveroo lunchbox, and a supply of Netflix. In fact, its load of sweaters and books comes in useful.

The temperature drops further. I can see the top of the mountain now, and its washing line of fluttering white prayer flags. Next, a wooden stake with a sign in white lettering on a dark green background: Dodeyora Buddhist Institute, Thimpu, Bhutan.

Take nothing but pictures, leave nothing but memories. Make your day beautiful. Monastic wisdom, Coldplay-style. And here at last is the monastic settlement nestling on the slope of the mountain. We look down on it from our summit. The two-story, whitewashed wooden houses form a community: a teaching quarter, the vice principal's quarters, a library, dormitories, and, in the center, a yellow-and-red building, which is the guesthouse. I notice the toilets seem to be in a separate block, and my heart sinks.

We rest for a while on a raised wooden platform, decorated with prayer wheels, or in this case, painted plastic bottles. I spin one with a goodwill thought: *Please, oh Lord, let me have my own lavatory.* Then I try again with a more high-minded wish about protecting Bhutan. I am trying to suppress the poison of personal desire and greed.

Finally, the last ascent past more messages of wisdom attached to trees. "Time is always with the person who has courage." And, "Some people dream of success while others work at it." And another one: "No beauty shines brighter than a good heart." This copywriter of homilies had good intentions and I am learning a principle of Buddhism, which is not to be so critical of others. Do not judge.

The entrance gates to the monastic college are colorful and friendly. Leaning against them is a motionless European woman with a reusable water bottle, deep in reflection. I register that it is surprising to see a Caucasian woman on her own here, in a male Buddhist monastery. I say hello, and she replies in accented English. When I look back, she is heading through a makeshift door into one of the cruder huts, which definitely does not have its own toilet or shower.

We meanwhile go into a guesthouse, leaving our shoes on the wooden porch. Inside it is decorated with burgundy layered rugs, low furniture, and bare light bulbs. The walls are papered in nursery yellow and orange patterns. Our bedroom has three single mattresses in it with blankets and covers that look like beach towels.

Lilacs and reds and blues, a cacophony of color. A heater keeps the room at an old-folks-home, toasty temperature, although when I try to open the little window an icy blast chills my hands.

Shortly afterward both the heat and the light blow out in a power cut. I am told that the monk who understands electrical systems is in class but he will have a look at the fuse box later. I grope my way in coat and socks to the bathroom, which currently has no running water, but does have the luxury of a broken-seated toilet.

The monks make do with a bank of washrooms. Next morning, the grass by the outside tap will be frozen.

We head for breakfast in the guesthouse dining room. If the furniture here is basic, it is not just because of monastic frugality. It is also because the monks have had to carry it up the mountain.

Two monks per sofa, twelve to heave up the transformer. A young monk glances at the bookcase, sighing. "Very heavy." The monks have an aesthetic dignity in their claret robes—you can see why Bertolucci loved Bhutan—but they are also just boys.

The teenagers assigned to serve us pile rice and soupy dahl onto hot plates on a table empty except for tea urns.

They have good English, thanks to the monastic education, and they can talk about Manchester United—comparing that team to their own matches on the abbot's football pitch. They don't meet enough people, or see enough places for any other cultural or geographical references.

They are pleased to be going home for their annual month's break in January. I ask them what they miss the most, being here away from home. "Food," grins one, speaking for teenagers around the world. Filling the bookshelf they hauled up the mountain path are Harry Potter books as well as volumes of Buddhist instruction. There is a signed football and some impressive football trophies. They have begun playing against the other monasteries. "It's war," says the more playful of the teenagers.

We settle into the floor-level sofas, drinking the canteen tea. The novice monks sit cross-legged against the wall, waiting for our questions, both studious and bantering. I ask the more gregarious one if he is prepared for his exams in a couple of weeks. He replies that his mind is so full of information that he has to pour a bucket of cold water over his head to calm it down.

He gives an account of his day: He is awake at 4:00 A.M. in the summer and 6:00 A.M. in the winter for prayers. Then it is study and more prayers until 10:00 P.M. The only distraction is the football pitch. There are no electronic games and no expectations of going anywhere. This clearing in the mountain forest is their world for about eleven months of the year. I wonder at the smallness of it, until I realize the limits of my own imagination. Just because they don't see the rest of the world does not mean that they cannot experience it. God is not visible, yet they have devoted their lives to him.

In the weakening, early-evening light, I discover perching places among the blue pines for solitary contemplation. My favorite has a view across the valley, the darkness broken only by sequin lights from Thimpu in the distance. Imagine living in this place—each day sitting on this tree stump on a forest ledge and watching the sun rise, lighting up the mountain, and then at the end of the day, seeing the silhouette of the mountains and valleys return against the blush-pink clouds.

The sun rises, the sun sets. I see neither of these things in the LED strip light of the office world. Yet this is the rhythm of the soul. The monks have a greater purpose. They sit on the mountain and chant in order to suppress the bad spirits that they believe bring suffering to humanity. They chant to see off ignorance, and anger, and greed, and pride. They chant for peace and harmony. In this region of Bhutan, I've seen a mural that depicts this purpose: In it a bird is perched on top of a rabbit, which is sitting on top of a monkey, which is in turn sitting on an elephant's back. The message is that if these four species can coexist, so should humanity.

As I wrap myself in a blanket against the icy gloom, a bell sounds and the claret-robed figures hurry up and down paths toward the wooden building arranged for evening prayers. I creep in after them and sit against the wall. The monks are assembled in two rows facing each other, bowing rhythmically as they start up the low murmur of liturgy. One of the boys yawns, another passes sweets from the improvised sleeve of his robe. It is cheekiness, not insolence. The chant is unbroken and by rote.

There are more prayers in the lit chamber above. Here a young boy of perhaps nine or ten sits in a throne chair, an older boy crouched at his side, who smiles as he passes him pages of liturgy. Two other boys sound long horns. Others hold up drums, which they strike with carved sprigs of wood. The native orchestra joins the voices in proclaiming the triumph of good.

I am starting to get pins and needles from my posture— sitting cross-legged for long periods separates the meditative folk from the rest of us. The chanting and the music are making me drowsy.

So I jump when a monk whispers in my ear that I have an invitation to see the principal of the monastery, who has the highest chalet on the mountain. I haul myself up and leave the chanting boys, their pure, incantatory voices echoing outside in the acoustics of the mountainside.

I climb the stone steps carved into the earth, my gloveless hands raw with winter cold. Above, a half-moon shines over the black-green forest. The perks of being principal turn out to be a television and a four-bar electric heater, but otherwise the room of the head monk is simple—rugs spread across the floor, a couple of sagging sofas.

The round-faced, bespectacled monk sitting opposite me cannot exactly remember his age, maybe thirty-eight, maybe forty, but he does remember becoming a monk at age thirteen. He had begged his mother to let him go and eventually she relented. Speaking in halting English, he tells me that, released from the world, he has been entirely happy ever since. The secret of happiness, he says, is to live harmoniously among nature, far from the city.

He practices monks medicine, which is a mix of the traditional and the scientific. There is the woodworm plant for congestion and the dandelion root for coughs and colds. He commends the mountain air as the best protection against illness.

Above all, he instructs me in the enlightening effect of an early start to the day. It is the one piece of monasticism that I am trained for. My news program starts at 6:00 A.M. and I am usually awake at 4:30 A.M. But I do not begin dawn in a transcendental state. Instead, it is a frenzy of news wires and Twitter. *What have we missed? What have we missed?* The monastic response is: nothing.

Then there is the mastery of equilibrium. He preaches acceptance as the route to happiness.

Envy and dissatisfaction are modern ailments. If you live in a mountain community, you are not constantly comparing yourself to others.

The principal has two rules. The first is to be happy with what you have; the second is to be kind to others. At this moment the door opens and the young Western woman I had seen earlier in the day at the gate peers round it apologetically. She is tall and athletic-looking in the doorway, with an open face and long, wavy fair hair.

She introduces herself as Anne and says in English that she has come from the Netherlands to learn about happiness from the principal. I tell her that I am writing about monastic wisdom, and am curious to know about her experience of it. I come as an observer; she is living here until Christmas. Anne stands in the center of the room, dominating it with her height. She is animated. She explains her background, a big job leading IT development for KLM, the Dutch airline. She was urban, faddy, keen on comforts. She was germophobic. Yet here she is, staying for a month with what we might politely call basic facilities.

"It was a culture shock," she smiles. For the first few days she concentrated hard on small pleasures, in the spirit of Buddhism. The sunlight over the forest. The friendliness of the monks. And then, after a few days, it clicked. She learned about the joy of silence. Above her room the tree sign proclaimed: "When a man knows the solitude of silence and joy of quietness he becomes free from fear and finds the joy of dharma—Buddha."

I am lagging far behind Anne in acceptance. That night, I sleep with all my clothes on because of the cold and cannot bring myself to use the broken toilet or the ancient basin. My amulet is my bottle of mineral water that I brought with me. I will the night to pass, remembering Saint John of the Cross and the dark night of the soul. If I lie still, with my eyes tightly shut, this will pass. Time in fact passes incredibly slowly if you follow this strategy. I can hear steady breathing from my husband in his single bed across the room. Is he actually sleeping?

The first light is a kind of miracle. From when I wake at 4:00 A.M., I keep bouncing up to check the window, and each time the dark is solid. Then it rises like a veil. I straighten out of bed, pull on a scarf and jacket, and open the door onto the porch. A cold mist envelops the peaks of the mountains, spreading like a spider's web over the pines and oaks and cypresses. The gong is being sounded for prayers. The echo of it mingles with the orchestra of the birdsong.

I kneel on a mat above the prayer house and look down on the valley. I see the claret figures and the backs of shaved heads scrambling down their paths, holding prayer books. The morning chanting begins, and as it does so, flocks of snow pigeons perform their synchronized acrobatics from mountain peak to mountain peak. Yellow-billed, blue-tailed magpies gather on a pine tree in front of me and chestnut-colored song thrushes alight on another. I spot a nutcracker.

The mist is now bowling across the trees but high above is a glimmer of blue. The effect of the light on the clouds is rose pink and dove gray. I gaze out at the roof of clouds and can just glimpse the higher peak, concealed behind it. You can trek from Paro to Thimpu along this ridge. The monastery seems like paradise.

After a breakfast of rice and chili and black tea, it is time to descend the path. Now I can see the silvery thread of the river and the blocks of houses below. There are so many types of plants on the route down; against the many shades of green are clusters of delicate white flowers. Even the pine cones are special—unusually large and lotus-like.

I turn back for one last look, but the monastic settlement has vanished. It disappears into the mist and then into the curve of the mountain. No one would know it was there.

Back in Thimpu, I sit under a cypress tree at the Astrology College and watch boy monks study their books. The act of study, on a patch of emerald grass, by a cleansing river, is a monastic tradition. Out of it grew the universities.

Then I wander back to the minibus past a group of men of working age, who have given up the day to an archery competition. This, said Tenzin, would be encouraged by their employees. You work to live, you do not live to work. Everything is balance here. That is happiness.

I have one more monastery to visit before we leave. Bhutan's most sacred site is Taktshang Goemba, Tiger's Nest Monastery. It is also one of the wonders of the world and, being Bhutan, it was closed to tourists until 2005. Once the tourists and pilgrims came, the monks left for higher land. They founded another monastery and now look across the mountain at the human ants and the mules who bring up supplies.

I can see Tiger's Nest from our guesthouse window. It is a white dot in the mountain. Guru Rinpoche is said to have meditated there for three years when he brought Tibetan Buddhism to Bhutan, and this is still how long monks have to practice meditation before they are considered fully trained.

The hermitage next to Tiger's Nest is where monks go on trial to see if they can cope with the isolation. The position looks impossible—Tiger's Nest clings to the rock face about three thousand feet (nine hundred meters) above the valley. It certainly appears too steep to climb, but the trail winds through familiar pine and Himalayan oak woods. My husband leads the hike, and I trail behind him, slipping on stones and stopping for breath. About two-thirds of the way up the mountain, I am becoming tired and grumpy. The water in my bottle is warm and my clothes are dusty. I can see my husband's springy hiking step far ahead of me and I curse him for his rebuking fitness.

Then, as I look down over the edge of the path, I spot the lichen, hanging in feathery lime-colored ribbons from the trees. It is like nature's hair, spreading itself over the valley. I have never seen anything like it. I am so entranced by the citrus purity of it that at first I do not register what is behind the trees. Then the lichen parts to reveal our first close-up view of the sheer rock and the crooked arrangement of white-washed walls and wooden roof that make up Tiger's Nest Monastery.

We continue up, up until we are eye level with Tiger's Nest but still cannot see how to cross the ravine. Then it becomes clear. There are hundreds of steps leading to a bridge and hundreds up the other side. Clear water gushes down the side of the rock. A redstart flies in front of me over the bridge. We have arrived.

At the entrance to the monastery, we are asked to hand in weapons, cameras, and phones, all categorized together. A group of pilgrims from Nepal and Bhutan are singing. Inside, we move from shrine to shrine, finding the entrance to the Guru Rinpoche cave, and finally a room of such magnificence that I am rooted to the spot.

In the center is a gigantic figure of Buddha representing longevity. At the far side, a figure of terror, Guru Rinpoche stamping on the evil spirits, one of whom looks slightly like a colonial Brit. A statue of a man and woman in tantric unity has, at its base, skulls, serpents, and heads representing the sins of desire, anger, ignorance, and pride.

In between the figures is a highly decorated frieze of wild animals, fire, and flowers. The room is empty, and I look out from it down on the forested valley and back at the incandescent gold figures. And I make the small sign of worship, hands to head, mouth, and chest. Something happens in that room. It is as if my spirit has flown from my body. I remember a distinguished American physicist named Brian Greene talking of the distinction between faith and science. He said that science was about searching to understand the outside world, the universe, while faith was an internal quest. In that room, I experience spirit and mountain.

As we start the trek down, we pass other pilgrims ascending in the midday heat; I call out encouragement. A local guide performs a yoga pose in the curved trunk of a tree above a twenty-three-hundred-foot (seven-hundred-meter) drop. Each step is hard but that is the nature of pilgrimages. Monks have an enhanced gravity, a liberation of faith. They are also protective deities on the mountain. A recent visitor who twisted her ankle was saved by monks who turned their robes into a stretcher.

My legs are liquid as I finish the last stretch to the base but there is a monastic cure for that. A bath heated by burning stones and scattered with the woodworm plant. I try to tempt my hiking husband into the bath, but he goes off instead on an evening walk. Virtue in others can be intensely annoying. From my outside bath, I look out through the steam, at the mountain and the cloudless sky.

I remember the words of Sogyal Rinpoche:

Reflect on this:

The realization of impermanence is paradoxically the only thing we can hold on to, perhaps our only lasting possession. It is like the sky, or the earth. No matter how much everything around us may change or collapse, they endure.

And those of Buddha:

This existence of ours is as transient as autumn clouds.

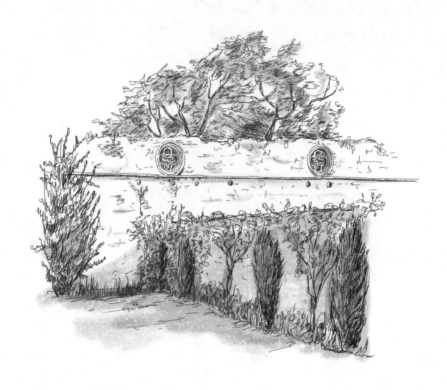

Chapter 6

SIMPLICITY AND THE INNER SILENCE

MARHAM ABBEY, NORFOLK

T he order of these chapters has changed from my original plan. Easter week was meant to have been spent in Salzburg, at the Nonnberg Abbey—otherwise known as the setting for *The Sound of Music*.

But then, in March 2020, the country went into lockdown, along with much of the rest of the world. Flights were halted, hotels closed. Monasteries continued in their customary state of self-isolation, and I was unable to reach them. Newspapers carried photographs of vats of beer and wine being emptied away. This was the London economy—bars and coffee shops. Farewell to my working life.

The existence that I was trying to escape in this book suddenly seemed unbearably delightful. I watched television scenes of dinner parties or concerts as if through a looking glass. My bank statements read like an historical archive. Soho House, Joe the Juice, Caffè Nero, Daniel Galvin, and, in the final days, Wigmore Street Pharmacy, Boots, Boots, Boots.

Like everyone else, I was separated from what and whom I knew and loved. Zoom entered the popular vocabulary. My younger son FaceTimed me from Hong Kong. He told me that he would not be coming home for his summer break because of the strict rule of quarantine.

My elder son sent me a photograph of my grandson, only twenty miles away, but beyond reach now. My daughter went into lockdown in London, the epicenter of the virus. Every family had a story to tell of separation.

Monasticism teaches that you can love and participate, while being absent. This was what I had to learn: to appreciate relationships in the abstract. To delight in the existence of others without physical engagement in their lives.

The government demanded that the population return to their homes: Mine was in Norfolk, in the remains of Marham Abbey. A monument to mortality and the futility of secular ambition. Henry VIII destroyed this monastery but could not destroy its meaning; perhaps because its endurance was based on acceptance of powerlessness.

The mood of the country was suddenly very Dark Ages. An intensive-care doctor on the radio described the strange, sticky properties of the virus. "I have not seen anything like this before—it is medieval."

I read an account of the impact of the Black Death by Henry Knighton, in 1348.

In this year and in the following one there was a general mortality of men throughout the whole world. It first began in

India, then in Tharsis, it came to the Saracens and finally to the Christians and the Jews. The King of Tharsis, seeing such a sudden and unheard of slaughter of his people began a journey to Avignon to propose to the pope that he would become a Christian, thinking that he might mitigate the vengeance of God upon his people. Then, when he had journeyed for twenty days he heard that the pestilence had struck among the Christians.

The Black Death raced through the monasteries: "There was not one of the English hermits left in Avignon."

As hospitals were filled with patients struggling for breath, the very act of breathing took on miraculous significance, and I thought of the Buddhist monks mastering the art of it. Stripped of all the glitter and ribbons of my life, I was content to be alone with the wall, breathing in and breathing out.

The book I read during this period was, of course, Hilary Mantel's *The Mirror & the Light*. The seizing of the monasteries by Thomas Cromwell to enrich the court of Henry VIII is a theme woven through the narrative. Yet Cromwell appreciated the spirit of the monasteries—and his preparation for death was monastic. He read and he prayed and tried to close the distance between life and death. The dark night of the soul was his reckoning.

● ● ●

Just before the lockdown was decreed, an archaeological dig took place in front of the wall. I had applied for planning permission to create a lily pond, in the spirit of Monet, as I had promised myself I would in the island of Naoshima, in Japan. First, the area had to be examined for historical significance.

At 8:00 A.M. on a bright spring Monday morning, a digger and three cheerful young folk in high-viz jackets arrived at the house. They were the archaeologists looking for evidence of remains in the soil above the chalk base, north of the abbey wall. They explained what they were searching for. Not treasure, but nuns' bones. On the whole, bodies are found in the east, the wealthier area near the chancery. But this was not a rich abbey. As I brought out mugs of tea, I experienced mixed feelings about the bones. On the one hand, I was curious; on the other, each skeleton would cost me seven hundred fifty pounds (about one thousand twenty-five dollars)—the cost of reburial.

The two young men were from Norfolk and Cambridge; their gregarious female assistant was a student from the West Country. The most serious, Tom, took meticulous notes and paced out lengths. The other young man, with Henry VIII coloring and a broad smile, took rippling pleasure in the digger throwing up ten-foot (three-meter) layers of topsoil, which then exposed the chalky base.

Nothing was revealed. They found one bone of no historical interest. I shrugged that it probably belonged to one of my missing husbands. The young woman laughed.

She disappeared later that day, but it was lockdown rather than nuns' bones that claimed her. Her parents drove through the night from Dorset to collect her. The following morning, the two men dug further and in earnest. They planted flags to signify potential. What they traced was a deep trench cut into the chalk rock. This was part of the precinct of the abbey. My house and garden, it turned out, were within the precincts. Around eight hundred years after this abbey brought Cistercian values to Norfolk, I was discovering its story.

On their last evening, the two men shared a cottage pie with us, at a social distance around the table as if we were in a baronial setting, which appeared awkward at the time but now seems familiar. They were all packed up to leave, their spades in their car, but they lingered. It was the pull of the wall. I watched them walk around it in the fading light, one last glance back, a further hesitation.

Then they were gone, but they left behind a hill of topsoil and a smaller pile of chalky earth. This I scattered on the path behind the wall. It fell right there, a moonlight-colored path, a shared history in the soil. We had been unearthing the structural facts of the abbey, but we were also renewing its meaning.

◦ ◦ ◦

I would describe the feelings I associated with the wall during those weeks of isolation as intense serenity and a sense of belonging. Most of all, I associated it with birdsong. The trees surrounding the abbey remains were full of birds—blackbirds, blue tits, finches, wrens, chiffchaffs, robins, rooks, and, descending from the wide skies, the first swallows. There was one thing I wished to learn in isolation: the distinctive differences in birdsong. On the first day I picked up the alarm call of the blue tits and the different whistles of the great tit. I wondered at the lung capacity of the tiny wrens. The busy sound of the chiffchaff will always remind me of this time, this period of death tolls and birdsong.

I learned to watch the sky. The Cloud Appreciation Society became personal and particular to me. The only patch of sky I was going to see for a while was this one. The dry spring weather created biblical luminosity—evening slices of blinding light between pink, navy, and gunboat-gray dusks. Sometimes the light widened panoramically, other evenings the sinking sun bequeathed "Norfolk lights" and fuchsia and orange patterns in the clouds.

The skies were wondrous during lockdown, observatory clear at night. Separated from loved ones, we looked up at the same supermoon.

A feature of coronavirus was that it struck the West just as nature was burgeoning. A doctor in New York named Qanta Ahmed wrote in *Spectator* magazine of the poignant contrast between the season and the terror and tiredness of critical care at the NYU Langone Hospital in Mineola.

> *In the rare moments when I can break away from the background noise of alarms and alerts that typify every intensive care unit, I hear birdsong. . . . Almost unnoticed, a New York winter entirely devoid of snow has given way to a cherry-blossomed spring.*

She quoted a poem by Pablo Neruda: "You can cut all the flowers, but you cannot keep spring from coming."

In the ash and horse chestnut trees to the west of the abbey wall, birds alighted on different branches and sang their hearts out as if it were Handel's *Messiah*. I could identify long-tailed tit, nuthatch, blackbird, robin, and song thrush.

Then their song was drowned out by the low-flight boom of the F35 stealth bombers on practice maneuvers, circling from the nearby RAF airbase. I was reminded of the faint, throat-catching BBC archive recording of the Lancaster bombers in the Second World War. What the recording unexpectedly picked up in the foreground was the song of a nightingale.

The *Today* program was being produced remotely, and I spent hours pacing the garden on Zoom. What were the latest death figures? What was the state of the prime minister's health? He had passed his dark nights in intensive care, watched over by nurses, whom he would later name with rising emotion. He described the National Health Service as the beating heart of the nation, powered by love. The country staked its identity on the principle of caring for the sick. A principle begun in its monasteries.

Indeed, St. Thomas' Hospital, where the prime minister was treated, grew out of a priory. A little museum nearby records early natural treatments. Meadowsweet, silver birch, and wormwood were the remedies monks might have offered. The monastery was dissolved in 1539—but later the hospital reopened.

Good Friday passed for the population indoors, without the warmth of sunshine or the caress of family and friends. It was a kind of mass imprisonment. A darkness fell over the land.

Yet here I was looking at the chalky limestone wall as a symbol of endurance and resilience. The wall is framed on one side by a yew, the oldest species of tree, pre-Christian, yet a feature of churchyards. Yews were planted in groves for religious worship in the Bronze Age. Then pre-Christian was absorbed by Christian. In medieval times Palm Sunday was known in Europe as Yew Sunday.

The tree's wood back then was prized for its flexibility—it was ideal for making longbows for archery. Yew weapons were used at the Battle of Agincourt in 1415, Henry V's great victory for the English over the French.

Another yew, nearer the house, was cut down before I lived here, to prevent it from blocking the light outside the bedroom window. Saddened by its stump, I grew clematis around it and planted a circle of blue anemones at its base. The birds then seeded a raspberry bush, which bandaged its trunk. Pinks and reds blended in profuse flowering. And birds gathered there. Blue tits nested. One day a nightingale settled. The wounded tree became cherished by nature.

The yew by the abbey wall, by contrast, is covered in needle leaves, richly dark. Sometimes the tree seems almost unified with my wall. They share the secrets of history. Looking out at the tree now, a verse from a poem by Sir Arthur Conan Doyle comes back to me, half remembered from childhood:

> *The bow was made in England;*
> *Of true wood, of yew wood,*
> *The wood of English bows,*
> *So men who are free*
> *Love the old yew tree,*
> *And the land where the yew tree grows.*

My Instagram feed has been refined since the virus began. I have ditched the celebrities and stuck with English Cathedral Windows and Norfolk Holkham Conservation—the light of the cross and the light of nature. Every evening for years, I have lit up the abbey wall with artificial light for a few hours so the village could look to its radiance for reassurance in the shadows.

I think of what Saint Thomas once called "the light of faith." If there is a divine truth beyond knowledge and reason, then my wall, bright behind the silhouette of the yew tree and the big dark sky, seems a testament to it.

⁕ ⁕ ⁕

This is what I have discovered about the history of Marham Abbey. It was founded in 1249 and dissolved in 1536. In its early years, it was under the control of the bishop of Ely, before being given to the Earl of Arundel and his wife, Isabel. After her husband's death, Isabel Aubigny took over the abbey for Cistercian nuns.

Marham was part of a small cluster of local monasteries. To the east of the paddock, across shooting land, was Pentney Abbey, which housed the Augustinian order. It is a finer ruin than Marham, with a notable flint gatehouse, and makes a point of its superiority by cloaking itself in scaffolding. Pentney was dissolved in 1537, the year after Marham. One amateur sleuth claimed a tunnel existed between Marham and Pentney. No one can find evidence of this, but it raised questions about the moral reputation of my nuns. Beyond are the ruins of Castle

Acre Priory, a Cluniac priory founded in 1089 and dissolved in 1537.

Norfolk was hit hard by Cardinal Wolsey's failure to persuade the pope to grant Henry VIII a divorce. From 1530 onward, Wolsey's replacement, Thomas Cromwell, helped the king demolish more than seven hundred Catholic monasteries, helping himself to their accounts.

The meekest went first. In 1535, the prioress and eight nuns at Marham Abbey signed the Deeds of Surrender of the priory to one of Cromwell's agents. It was valued at thirty-three pounds and thirteen shillings. It has a rather slighting description in the catalog of Norfolk monasteries:

> *Being of little wealth or status, in 1536 the monastery was in the first wave of closures during the Dissolution of the Monasteries and was reportedly in considerable disarray, with the inhabitants accused of disreputable behavior.*

Of some fifty-nine abbeys and priories in medieval Norfolk, around twenty are now razed to the ground, and a handful have been reduced to a mere pile of stones. Marham is one up from the stones. Elsewhere, there are well-preserved relics. King's Lynn has Greyfriars Tower. Then there is the hamlet of Babingley, with the ruin of Saint Felix's parish church. This was said to be the spot where Felix of Burgundy brought Christianity to East Anglia in AD 603. The English Benedictine monk Bede praised Felix for rescuing East Anglia from "longstanding unrighteousness and unhappiness."

About thirty miles from Marham is Walsingham with the imposing remains of the Priory of Our Lady of Walsingham. Walking through the woods beyond Castle Acre near my house, I have stumbled across pilgrims, holding their crosses aloft, on the route to Walsingham. Coronavirus has hit religious gatherings hard. The woods are empty of pilgrims now.

The list goes on: Thetford Priory, founded in 1103 by Cluniac monks; Binham Priory, a Benedictine priory founded in 1091; Beeston Priory near Sheringham, Coxford Priory near Fakenham, Saint Faith's Priory, Langley Abbey. Norfolk is a county of monastic ruins, a civilization dissolved, the monastic principles of healing and education transferred to other institutions.

Saint Radegund's Priory, Cambridge, dissolved in 1496, went on to become Jesus College, Cambridge, courtesy of John Alcock, bishop of Ely. Monks and nuns took up work in hospitals. Through universities and infirmaries, the traditions of learning and the unconditional care of the sick survived. But the communities of contemplative spirituality were gone.

I often walk to Castle Acre from my house, via the monastic remains of nearby West Acre, through woodland, past a mill house, and along a trout stream so limpid that I can see the rust- and mustard-colored pebbles on its sandy floor, and the reflection of the birch trees on the banks. The path continues through marshland, in which swans slip through the grasses and reeds, and on to a field of cattle surrounded by hawthorn hedge—a sloping medieval landscape, at the bottom of which is Castle Acre.

There is a reference to it in Hilary Mantel's book, in a communication between Thomas Cromwell and Lord Norfolk.

Lord Norfolk writes: "I am so short of money I shall have to sell land and that comes hard. For God's sake put some abbeys my way."

He, Cromwell, almost rips up the letter in a rage. "Has he not just made a bargain with the duke for the abbey at Castle Acre? Can nothing sate the brute?"

Castle Acre is of the same period as my wall but survives in grander and so more melancholy outline. It looks unearthly from a distance, a scene from a holy grail, glimpsed behind the gateway of an ancient oak tree. But on approach, through the cattle, the irregular-shaped stones become cogent. A low wall, a central nave and cloisters, an upper floor. Yes, you see why Lord Norfolk had his eye on Castle Acre.

It housed Cluniac monks, originally from Burgundy in France, who believed God should be worshipped in splendor. The prior's lodgings survive, gracious in the imagination.

When Castle Acre Priory was dissolved, the monks were forced out, and the estates passed to Edward Coke, whose descendant, the Earl of Leicester, owns the land today. The monastic and the pastoral here create a landscape of solace.

My elder son leased a pheasant shoot from the Leicester estate last year, and I watched the wintry scene of a line of guns and twitching dogs at the edge of turnip fields. At lunch, in a makeshift lodge, the party of farmers in tweeds and thick socks discussed crops and taxes. Not so much had changed since the sixteenth century.

The priory lies in the palm of Castle Acre, among oak trees and horse chestnuts with sturdy Tudor girths. The splotches of sunlight between the battleship-gray clouds cast shadows of the towers, nave, and cloisters and sparkle across the oak leaves.

The twenty-five monks who lived in the priory would pray, bind books, tend the land, or look after the beehives. Bees are still associated with monasteries. I brought back matchless white honey from Ethiopia, the land of monasteries.

Medicinal gardens are part of monastic lore. Castle Acre Priory based its garden on a ninth-century monastery in Switzerland. The beds were divided into culinary, medicinal, strewing, and decorative growing areas, a bay tree standing at the center. There were also old apple trees: Ashmead's Kernal, Sheep's Nose, and Coeur de Boeuf.

The names of the medicinal plants have an incantatory sound to them: comfrey, lady's mantle, peony, bugle, pennyroyal, and thyme. Comfrey, also known as "knit bone," is said to heal wounds and burns. If I am to understand the monastic use of herbs and plants, it will probably be through the work of Nicholas Culpeper, a seventeenth-century astrologer physician who set up a practice in Spitalfields, London, and left a legacy of hundreds of herbal remedies.

He might not have been able to explain the science, but the plants helped heal his patients. For this reason, he pleaded with the medical establishment to include empiricism in their judgments. It takes monastic modesty to use medicinal herbs without making any grand claims for them.

In his book *Herbal Guide to Radiant Health*, Nicholas Culpeper recommended lady's mantle, also known as "dewcup," for the dew gathered in its leaves. The dew was said to represent "Our Lady's tears." It was used to treat painful periods and even endometriosis. An herbal drink of Our Lady's tears sounds comforting to me.

Thyme was the real wonder drug, soothing the stomach, easing sciatica, and purging the body.

Now, as the shelves of pharmacists are stripped of acetaminophen, hand sanitizers, and tissues, the government is spending billions and using every sinew to find ways of warding off coronavirus. After a couple of months, they come up with vitamin D.

I am beginning to appreciate the properties of herbs for well-being. I am drinking from jugs of water with a sprig of mint, and adding thyme and rosemary from my newly planted herb garden to chicken soup. As for mental health, what is better than peaceful seclusion and the presence of butterflies—painted ladies, the common blue (the modesty of its name belies the powder-blue perfection), the small whites with orange tips?

Before the brutal end to their community, the Cluniac monks lived well here. I can picture them at work on their books or among their plants. My Cistercian nuns, who wore white, were keener on discipline and labor.

◦ ◦ ◦

Back at home, looking out at the wall from the landing window, I can see a gray mare, a chestnut stallion, and a comical Shetland pony in the field beyond it. The farmer keeps racehorses for Fakenham, although nobody is racing now.

Horse people take a robust view of health—the last great public event just before lockdown was Cheltenham races. A right-wing hunting friend of mine wrote afterward that many of his friends were felled by Cheltenham. Being brave and merry was not enough to save you from the virus.

Beneath the earth, where the horses graze and swish their tails, lie the bones of the community of women in white. It is not clear what precisely the charges were against my Cistercian nuns, and I hope that it was not the sisterhood in disarray that drew me to buy the land. There is some local folklore. A highwayman was operating in the district, and many travelers, having been robbed and beaten, awoke to find themselves at Marham Abbey, being cared for by a Sister Barbara and her nuns. Gratefully, they donated gifts and money to the abbey. Only later did they discover that they had been duped, and that Sister Barbara and the highwayman were in business together. The last abbess at Marham recorded, in 1511, was named Barbara Mason.

But this may be Cromwellian slander or a not unfamiliar diminishing of the female contribution. There were only two Cistercian nunneries in medieval England, one in Dorset and mine in Marham. Tales were told of them as if they were girls' boarding schools. Sister Barbara seizes the imagination. One relative who stayed at my home claimed to have met her in one of my bedrooms. I watch the wall night after night and have never seen a silhouette other than that of a deer, or a cry that was not that of a tawny owl or a pheasant.

There were no stains cast on Sister Barbara's predecessor, Joan Heighham, 1486–1501. She was exemplary at book-keeping. I know this because her set of figures for one year are recorded in the archives.

Rent of assise for the Abbey Manor	*12 pounds, 16 shillings and 8 pennies*
Assise for Manor of Denhams	*1 pound and 3 shillings*
Assise for Manor of Besthorp	*3 shillings*
For farm of the rectory Dydlington	*53 shillings and 4 pennies*
Hackford	*Nothing, it being the year in the hands of the vicar by way of augmentation*
Stow Bedon	*53 shillings and 4 pennies*
Pension out of Rockland	*13 shillings and 4 pennies*
Land at Wymondham, Carlton, Fourhow, and Kimberly	*40 shillings*
For land in Kentford, Needham, and Gasely	*26 shillings and 8 pennies*
For land in Heringwell	*16 shillings*
For land in Shouldham	*10 shillings and 2 pennies*
For corn sold	*11 pounds, 9 shillings and 11 pennies*

For wool sold	*1 pound, 6 shillings and 8 pennies*
Hides and skins of cattle out of which was 8s for 12 ox hides	*9 shillings*
Agistment of sheep	*28 shillings*
Agistment of cows	*22 shillings*
Received from Leonard Cotton for his board	*26 shillings*
For the watermill	*Nothing*

Total received for this year: 46 pounds 18 shillings and 1 penny

This grand sum would have been turned over to Thomas Cromwell, after the Act of Supremacy. I can imagine Joan, writing by candlelight after the labors of the day—looking up at the wall, as I look to it now.

Scattered beyond the wall are a few faintly carved blocks of stone in the brambles, like a parochial Ozymandias. There is a carving of a hooded head, which could be a monk or a crusader. An aesthetic friend, who used to run English Heritage, suggested that we make a table out of these two blocks. A local builder arrived enthusiastically with a sack barrow to move the stone. The barrow dramatically broke, the stones fell. We returned them to their original site.

We did save one slab of stone, and a local blacksmith made a stand for it to make it into a bench. It sits underneath the circle of yew trees on the front lawn of the house, with sweet-smelling verbena bushes on either side. When I look at the wall in profile from the distance of the lawn, it looks more fragmentary. Some of its foundation stones are missing and ivy rings the window rims like sunken shadows. It lacks mass, looking sweetly transient after all.

We cannot dig the field because the abbey is a scheduled monument. But we have a drone view. The scruffy mounds of grass take clear shape from the sky. A high altar for the nuns and a church for the lay people. A cloister, refectory, kitchen, lay house, chapter house, and outer parlor.

Five or six times a year, someone will knock on the door—a student or an amateur historian, wanting to do a project on the wall. Amateur history is the great British hobby. Then come the metal detectorists, who have so far found nothing. I have a blue folder, the sum of investigations into the wall, by the country's enthusiasts.

Thanks to the public, I learned for instance that Communion was served in pewter, not gold. And that the priory kept sheep and pigs, and planted so many cherry trees that the village became known as Cherry Marham until the nineteenth century. The Cistercians built their monasteries in remote places so they could avoid all the distractions of life. The twelfth-century historian William of Malmesbury called the order "the surest route to heaven." Lockdown is not the same as monasticism but both involve a forcible removal from social structures and both allow for simplicity and contemplation.

The routines of my day are fundamentally altered. The flight from the urban network to rural isolation is existential. A journalist friend, a man in his sixties, writes to me:

I am in the country, have been here for weeks because I was spooked early by COVID. I write all day, garden, and walk. Never see anyone. The countryside is extraordinary—no traffic, no machines, no jet trails, no boats. I went to cut hazel bean sticks and it struck me that for the first time we are hearing the countryside as Wordsworth did.

While my friend looks to Wordsworth, I look up the teachings of Pythagoras, the ancient Greek philosopher who proposed a harmonious existence. His seventeenth-century biographer, Thomas Stanley, gave an account of the daily routine of the disciples of Pythagoras:

These men performed their morning walks by themselves and in such places where they might be exceeding quiet and retired. These were temples and groves and other delightful places. For they thought it was not fit they should speak with anyone till they had first composed their souls and fitted their intellect—and that such quiet was requisite for the composure of their intellect. For as soon as they arose, to intrude among the people they thought a tumultuous thing.

After they had studied awhile, they went to their morning exercises. The greater part used to anoint themselves and run races, the fewer to wrestle in orchards and groves.

At dinner they used bread and honey. The time after dinner they employed in political affairs.

As soon as the evening came, they betook themselves again, not singly as in their morning walks, but two or three walked together. After their walks, they used baths and washing. Then

*they went to supper that they might end it before the Sun was
set. After supper they offered libations, then had lectures. These
and all the other actions of the day they contrived in the morning
when they woke, and examined before they slept.*

They walked, they ate simply, they learned. It was a medieval
existence; it suddenly feels a contemporary answer. About thirty
miles from Marham is a Carmelite nunnery named Quidenham,
which I have visited twice. I feel its proximity keenly. The imaginative empathy is partly because I know what the nuns are
doing at different times of day. Nothing changes, and it is the
fixed exterior that allows the expanding interior.

The Carmelites owe their name to Mount Carmel in the
Holy Land. This was a ridge on the edge of the Mediterranean
Sea, on the Bay of Haifa in Israel. The juxtaposition of sea and
land was compared to the relationship between heaven and
earth. Mount Carmel is not quite of this world.

They were hermits and then pilgrims, with a particular
concentration on the birth and death of Christ. The author
of *The Carmelite Way*, John Welch, sums up the appeal of the
mountain, the sea breeze, and the clarity of being: "It freed
hearts that had been anxious about many things. The oratory in
the midst of the cells invited them to find a centre in the midst
of their lives."

Warfare claimed the Middle East, then as now, and the
Carmelites traveled to Cyprus, Sicily, France, and England. The
order began to decline in the fifteenth century, but in 1452 a
papal bull allowed nuns to enter it (having been men only before

this). The first communities of women were in the Netherlands and Florence.

In sixteenth-century Spain, the Carmelite nun, Teresa of Avila, had a vision of restoring the hermit tradition of Mount Carmel. She believed solitude was the most important condition for enlightenment. She also made a vexing demand for a small community of women, that everyone should be loved. She was helped in her reform of the Carmelite order by Saint John of the Cross.

He believed that human desire can never be satisfied. All the wealth and distraction and stimulation in the world only increase anxiety and discontent. Peace comes with a silent interior. The need to withdraw is a deep principle of the Carmelites.

The tension between the distractions of urban life and inner peace have been experienced for centuries. In 1270, a French Carmelite prior general named Nicholas wrote a letter, known as "The Flaming Arrow," addressed to his brethren, urging a retreat from the cities and citing the blessings of the desert.

> *In the desert all the elements conspire to favor us. The heavens, resplendent with the stars and planets in their amazing order, bear witness by their beauty to the mysteries higher still. The birds seem to assume the nature of angels, and tenderly console us with their gentle caroling. The mountains too, as Isaiah prophesied "drop down sweetness" incomparable upon us and the friendly hills "flow with milk and honey" such as is never tasted by the foolish lovers of this world.*

He went on to praise the trees, the breeze, the sunshine. By contrast, city life was pestilent.

In the city, the elements teem with such corruption that you too are contaminated and directly infected. . . . For melodious bird-song, you hear men and women brawling . . . for the scent of fragrant flowers, your nostrils drink in pestilential draughts of the intolerable stench of depravity.

The great escape from London during the coronavirus pandemic seems a testament to the beliefs of Nicholas. I have made my life in the city. For the five years until 2017 that I edited the *Evening Standard,* I spent every evening in theaters or restaurants or at parties. When Boris Johnson was mayor, he invited me to the London Olympics, and it felt as if it were the center of the world. The coronavirus has seen off globalization and political hubris, not to mention big public gatherings; at least for the time being. In its place comes an appreciation of looking after others, of reading, of openness to nature, and of humility. Self-isolation has provided a route to clarity.

The question is, what does it mean to live a full life? Teresa of Avila teaches that a life lived well demands a surrender of self rather than a gratification of desire. I think of this while listening to a man with terminal cancer on the radio, thwarted by the lockdown from seeing his children. He spoke, with a sob, of separation and then was asked by the interviewer what gave him pleasure. He said that it was watching the changes in nature in his garden, and hearing the birdsong. His act of contemplation had been planting beans in his allotment even if they outlived him. A vale of suffering and green shoots.

This, at least, is the teaching of the Carmelites, but what is it like to live their life? Does it feel like an isolated existence?

Quidenham is the Norfolk nunnery made famous by the surprising television celebrity, the late Sister Wendy Beckett. When Sister Wendy was asked what the other nuns thought of her television career as an art historian, which brought her fame and travel, she answered: "They feel sorry for me." The values we uphold are the opposite of those of the nunnery. Silence and selflessness are their means to deepest joy.

Quidenham is about an hour's drive from Marham toward Norwich, the cathedral city of Norfolk. There are a couple of hermit guesthouses within the nunnery's two hundred acres, and when I first inquired, it turned out these were booked months in advance. Isolation is the modern luxury.

It was a sullen, bitingly cold day in November when I made my first visit, and the car rocked in the wind as I drove through Thetford woods. I went past bleak stretches of brown fields and trees, with rural attractions of paintballing and race tracks, and Thai lady massages. Past timber merchants and industrial storage, and then down a country lane through a village and past a sign for a hospice. The children's hospice stood in a peaceful, wooded, tidy hamlet. Its Christmas lights were shining but there were no sounds of children.

Beyond it was the Carmelite monastery, also silent and without movement. It is a graceful red-brick house, facing open countryside. I found a sign for reception and pressed the buzzer. A clipped woman's voice instructed me to come in from the cold.

The reception was a plain room with a red-tiled floor. In the center of it were four small wooden chairs around a table, on which stood a statue of the Virgin Mary and child. There was a library shelf of books with titles such as *Living in Mystery, Living Water, The Way of Perfection, Between Earth and Sky*, and the works of Teresa of Avila and John of the Cross. In the corner was a dollhouse-style replica of the monastery, with tiny details of the nuns in their brown-and-white habits, their prayer books in the choir stalls, and a miniature organ. It was made by a villager whom the nuns had helped.

From the open door to the parlor came a sing-song voice and a clatter of cups: Sister Stephanie who, although Quidenham is a closed order, had agreed to talk to me for an hour before vespers, the evening prayers. She appeared from her side of the bench with some crockery and offered me black tea or coffee. I took the Nescafé.

Sister Stephanie has large blue eyes, a narrow nose, a generous mouth, and beautiful clear skin. She combines a light, quick-to-laughter manner with core stillness. Despite her beguiling youthfulness, Sister Stephanie was actually fifty-one years old. She entered the monastery at age thirty-three, leaving behind not only her human resources job at Aviva, or Norwich Union as it then was, but also her mother and brother and the life she might have lived. Sister Stephanie's vocation crept up on her. At York University, where she read Economic History, she asked a German exchange student what she planned to do and the young woman answered: "I am going to be a Carmelite nun."

In her twenties, Stephanie took on more responsibilities at work, did voluntary work, had plenty of friends. She was busy but fundamentally restless and lonely. She described it as having too many personalities. Then she experienced a jolt of understanding, a glimpse of a life of contemplation. She described the moment as brief, intense, profound. She heard an inner voice, crystal clear, asking her to follow a vocation as a Carmelite nun, and she understood that the voice would not be heard again.

So she swapped her old way of life for a contemplative order, and has never left the monastery except for medical appointments and visits. In her old life, she would be preparing for the office Christmas party. Here, she works, reads, prays.

These are some of the lessons she has learned. First, the meaning of being an integrated rather than a divided self. Stephanie's eyes widened at the concept of social media, which dawned just as she retreated. She observed that people were constantly creating, deleting and re-creating themselves. They experimented and paraded in front of an audience. There was an addictive need to be noticed.

She, by contrast, has gone through a surrender of self and a transformation into transparency. She said the process was painful and embarrassing but ultimately liberating.

Second, she has learned to live among a small community forever. Outside the monastery, people struggle with relationships, especially marriages, despite society, entertainment, distraction. She must love a group of other women, and mostly in silence. It is self-discipline and prayer that transform sensation, impulse, and feelings of irritation or envy into contemplative love.

During the lockdown, cases of domestic violence have soared and mental health experts have advised on emotional release and how to access help lines. Sister Stephanie has long since learned to live alongside others without the roots of family or sex or economic and cultural self-interest. The lessons of toleration turn out to be fellow feeling. They are together so they must care for each other.

A third lesson is understanding the meaning of being alone. Stephanie pointed out kindly that we are all alone; it is just that most of us try frantically to disguise it. Confronting it is a reconciliation of life and death. Her guiding text was *The Shattering of Loneliness*, by Erik Varden, the abbot of Mount Saint Bernard Abbey in Leicestershire, the only Trappist house in England. He wrote of the harmony of silence.

Stephanie had a kind of meditative energy as she described the meaning of silence. She said that living in silence gave her a sense of the "movement and meaning of time." It deepened relations with others. She said that the nuns communicated at a deep and noncurious level. There is no small talk because there is no need. They need never ask: "What did you do today?"

She was concerned by the instantaneous quality of outside life. It is communication without thought or compassion. It is, she said, gratification rather than gratitude. It is not that Stephanie demands external silence. She is used to the sound of low-flying American planes from the local airbase. She can hear the race track. It is the constant stimulation of chat, the jabber of news that prevents thinking.

"I have never been bored here," she said. I described to her the glories of Fountains Abbey in Yorkshire and she was luminously interested, but did not make the connection that the rest of us would. She did not say "I *must* go there."

The contemplative life is internal. For Sister Stephanie, it is fulfilling. The nuns work diligently—Teresa of Avila instructed the Carmelites to work for a living and at Quidenham they make greeting cards and soaps. They pray. Sister Stephanie repeats a phrase used by the former head of Goldman Sachs, Lloyd Blankfein. She was trying, she said, to do "God's work." He meant creating wealth, she meant owning nothing.

I asked if there was monks medicine at Quidenham and she nodded. There is the garden and the soap, which is remedial. But she said: "If I think about being a Carmelite, I think of the veil being drawn back between eternity and time. It is learning to be joyful—and unafraid. Unafraid to be human." As I left, I offered my hand to shake but she took both my hands gently. It was the most discreet of blessings.

Almost a year later, I returned to Quidenham. This time, I stayed in their guest room, the hermitage. It is intended for those considering joining holy orders, but increasingly people on the outside are asking to book it for at least forty-eight hours of solitude and reflection. The great contemporary quest for peace of mind.

I had been that day at a social lunch—one of my son's shooting lunches on the edge of Castle Acre. It was cheerful and exuberant—dogs and children weaving their way around the table and under it. The group were baffled that I should be leaving this family scene to drive for an hour to stay in a monastery.

The monastery was dark, but a bell was tolling. I let myself in through the wooden door and a caretaker told me that vespers was taking place in the chapel. I crept up the narrow steps to an anteroom, from which there was a view across to the pews.

There were the nuns in their white capes and brown habits. There were psalms, and hymns, and prayers. They lit their candles in darkness, so that they resembled a Vermeer painting. An elderly nun at the end of the pew tried to hold hers with a shaking hand, and was helped by a neighbor. As the service ended, the nuns took off their white mantles and filed out in their dark robes. I remembered then what silence sounds like.

A door opened and a nun approached me. She was Sister Lesley, originally from Seattle, and she had come to show me to my guest room. It was outside the main nunnery, and it was dark and raining as I followed her down the path. I asked her how she found the British winters and she said it was not so different from Seattle. It was everything else about her life in a religious order that was dramatically different.

My room had a little kitchenette, a shower, a single bed, a desk, a bookshelf, and a cross. I had imagined it would be like a sixth-form boarding school room and it was. But without my possessions. I had brought a hot-water bottle and my own pillow and some sweet-smelling face creams. These might be my red lines if I were to stay at this nunnery. I took out my phone to tell the family WhatsApp about my room. No service. This was a kind of rehab for life.

Sister Lesley told me that one of the nuns would like to see me, in the visitors' room. It was Sister Stephanie. I was so pleased to see her, with her skin still glowing—and her smile wide.

I told her about the monasteries I had so far visited. She was animated and curious without any trace of envy. I told her about my room and asked about the other occupants. She told me about a doctor who was considering religious orders, and two women who had started to clear out a lot of possessions, which had led to them contemplating an interior purity. I asked her about the necessary conditions for potential nuns. How do you know when it is right?

She said there were first the precluding conditions. Those with depression are not admitted, since the intensity of self-examination and solitude required by Carmelites may damage a person suffering from depression as well as the community of nuns. Those with debts must clear them first. Those with dependents, children or parents, are warned against entering. And, for now, no transgender nuns. Ecclesiastical law recognizes the gender on your birth certificate only.

The Catholic Church now decrees that it takes nine years to become a fully-fledged nun. It used to be less, but these days it is harder to reach the necessary state of enlightenment. People arrive with the baggage of modernity, complicated lives, trauma, expectations.

The Carmelite experience is a casting off. Sister Stephanie said a sense of both humility and value takes some time to get right. She told me about the elderly nun among them who had been fearful of her failing health until she remembered a lesson from Saint Paul and said to Sister Stephanie: "Christ is happy with me as I am."

This was the method of Sister Wendy Beckett, who is buried here. Sister Stephanie said Sister Wendy had had no interest in her own celebrity; she had pointed instead to art, which she thought was a route to faith. Look there!

I asked Sister Stephanie about the medieval teachings of monks—that they should aim to reach a state of such peace that they could die without fear, because they had been preparing for it all their monastic life. She explained that I was talking about completion, which is the rhythm of the Carmelite day. Just before compline, the final prayers of the day, there is a short period of self-examination, in order to clear your conscience. The final prayer of compline is "Lord grant me a quiet night and a perfect end." Sister Stephanie said she sleeps like a log after this.

This is the gift of retreat.

She clasped my hands again in hers and wished me a good night. I returned to my room; the silence here was much deeper than I am used to. No cars passing, no television, no voices. I picked up my phone, I remembered, I put it away. I started to feel the beginnings of interior silence. There were no distractions. I thought of my day. There was quite a lot to examine in my conscience. I thought of priorities; how much did the excitement of political news really matter? I thought of my family and loved ones, wishing them well with the calmness of solitude. I did not require anything of them tonight.

❦ ❦ ❦

The bell the next morning sounded at 4:30 A.M. and then again at 5:00 A.M. These were *Today* program hours but without booze and social media. It made a big difference. I rose and looked at the little garden and the shadow that was becoming a tree. The lights were on at the nunnery as prayers began. I shut the front door quietly, carrying my laptop, phone, and pillow—essential props for me, unnecessary for the nuns.

I was reminded of Sister Wendy Beckett's response to the modern quest for self-fulfillment. It was not about me. The dawn repose of the nunnery is aided by their simple prayer: "Christ, have mercy upon me." I kept the car lights low as I passed the apparently unoccupied children's hospice, back over the pretty, old brick bridge, past the long wall back onto the main road to King's Lynn. The sky was black in front of me, but there were streaks of light behind—the dark night was passing into dawn.

By the time I saw the monastic wall in front of my house, the sky was a Norfolk canopy of gray white. It was 7:00 A.M. when I crept back into bed with my husband, back into my old life. I liked my bath, with its particular oils; I liked my breakfast of tea, blueberries, yogurt, and granola rather than the loaf of bread left out for me by the nuns. I was too attached to worldly pleasures after all, but I did not forget the nuns: "It is not about me" makes things much, much happier.

For some months, I was absorbed by the politics of Brexit. I decided on a change of career and gave in my resignation. A grandson was born, still a source of awe and wonder for me. But when the lockdown happened, when I became properly acquainted with my abbey wall, the face of Stephanie and the memory of vespers returned to me.

The lessons of Saint John of the Cross were designed for self-isolation: "Speaking distracts one, while silence and work recollects and strengthens the spirit." Here in lockdown I could glimpse Sister Stephanie's journey: The less we have around us, the less we need.

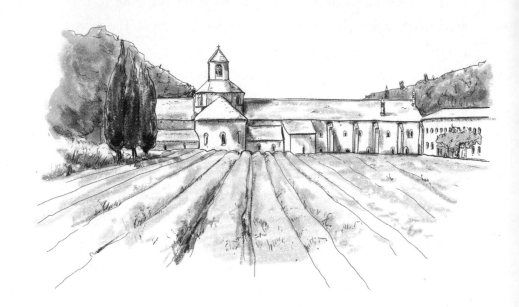

Chapter 7

TRUTH AND SILENCE

ABBAYE NOTRE-DAME DE SÉNANQUE

T ruth, like light, wounds the feeble sight, and at first excites a movement of repulsion. But though it may be impeded in its solemn promulgation at first, nothing can extinguish its brilliancy nor hinder its final triumph through the world.

This is Saint Bernard's Apology.

In July, I leave a fearful kind of isolation for a joyful one. I am going to the Luberon in southern France with my husband, son, daughter-in-law, and grandson. It is the first time since lockdown that I can hold my grandson's muscle-less, cherubic form and breathe him in. I watch him poised between delicious curiosity and the shock of discomfort and disappointment. He grabs my face mask as a comedic game. The pandemic is just the world he was born into.

We are staying in a former convent at the top of a hill along a pilgrim's route. The thick limestone walls offer security against the mistral wind and the temptations or pestilence of towns. During an outbreak of the plague in the seventeenth century, nuns took sanctuary at a convent in these hills.

Looking far down over wooded hills and patchwork hay-strewn fields I can see only the spire of the nearest village of Saint Michel. At night, the velvet-black sky is ablaze with stars. The earth is silent beneath. Nations may be anxious or sorrowful but the heavens are bright.

In the morning, when the cockerel wakes us even before the baby, we all walk while it is still cool. Wild-grass paths lead to tracks opening onto views of foothills and distant mountain ranges. Everything is soft and layered so that evening is a curtain of gauze, which drops to reveal the starry night with a parade of comets and satellites. On the old oaks and birches hang green-gray lichen as intricate as coral.

I am learning to adjust my sight to the palettes of sunrises and sunsets, darkness into light and light into darkness. I am also preparing myself for an inner quietness, for I have booked in at the Abbaye Notre-Dame de Sénanque, near Gordes, about an hour from this house. It is a Cistercian monastery, like my fragment of garden wall once was.

I had feared that the monastery would cancel my visit; everyone is jittery about a second wave of COVID and quarantine rules are being tightened.

A Trappist order of Cistercian monks hidden in a valley, surrounded by lavender fields, is statistically unlikely to encounter COVID. The monks have no need of company and are sustained by the vegetables they grow. If ever there were a time to seal themselves completely from the outside world, it is now.

But when I email to check, I am told that I am welcome to stay. I type rather than call because I do not imagine that picking up the phone appeals even to the administrative staff.

It is the prospect of silence that most intrigues me. As lockdown starts to lift, we are relearning the rhythms of conversation. I talk incessantly to my grandson, who is starting to follow what I am saying. Some words fill him with mirth. *Canoe* is one. *Huawei* is another. I am encouraging him to speak so that he can be fully human.

But Trappists believe that talking disturbs inner contemplation. It is in silence that they experience heavenly peace. They aspire to be less human.

The Cistercian order at Sénanque is based on the teachings of the twelfth-century monk Saint Bernard of Clairvaux. He entered the Abbey of Cîteaux in Dijon in 1113, aged twenty-three, with the words: "If thou beginnest, begin well." Some of us blunder through life instead, but I hope to learn to recognize virtue when I see it.

Saint Bernard had been a scholastic child and a fastidious teenager. When he was nineteen, he was so determined to resist an encounter with a beautiful woman that he jumped into a frozen pond and was finally dragged out almost senseless. He took the long view and found worldly passions distracting. He said: "Life is short, the world passes away, and you will pass away before it. Why not cease to love what will soon cease to exist?" This is the early detachment practiced by monks, the serenity of separation.

So he chose hardship, toil, and above all prayer as a means of liberating himself from the pleasures of life. His distinction was between pleasure and joy. Saint Bernard left Cîteaux to found a community at Clairvaux Abbey in 1115, where monks were bound to the strict Benedictine rules of the sixth century, which were to pray and work. But the Benedictines had slackened over the centuries, and the Church had become rather too merry. The thirteenth-century Archbishop Odo of Rigaud was scandalized by what he saw when he visited rural clergy in Normandy, as he writes in his diary:

> *Feb 1248, We visited the deanery of Brachi near Saint Just. We found that the priest of Ruiville was ill famed with the wife of the stone carver and by her is said to have had a child; also he is said to have many other children; he does not stay in his church, and he rides around in a short coat.*

So Saint Bernard led the new order of Cistercians into the hair-shirt existence of sacrifice. They lived apart from the secular world so that they could do penance for the rest of us.

These first Cistercians grew to 160 houses across Europe, and Saint Bernard was in time called upon to settle the legitimacy of popes and the rightful claimant to the German imperial throne. Unfortunately, he also inspired the disastrous Second Crusade, from 1147 to 1149, during which French troops under Louis VII were defeated by the Turks.

Saint Bernard later described the Crusade as "the season of disgrace" but consoled himself that the epic casualties had at least redeemed the troops and brought heaven closer to them. The Crusades, and the obsession with Jerusalem, are part of monasticism, for better or for worse.

"Hail, holy land! Land of human sorrows and divine mercies," wrote Saint Bernard.

He died back at his beloved cloister of Clairvaux in Burgundy, in 1153, aged sixty-three. Alas, the monastery is now ruins, a new civic building in its place. I cannot trace my own monument to the Cistercians back to its inspiration.

But in the Cistercian Abbey of Notre Dame de Sénanque, I can get close to the life of Saint Bernard. Prayer is the structure and meaning of the day. It is a life of separation from the world.

It was established by a dozen monks in 1148, seven years before Bernard's death, and according to a local guide book, he influenced the site and the design of the monastery—a secluded wooded vale, a building of limestone and slate, the semicircular church model of Clairvaux. It is described as the architecture of silence.

It is not too high—spires were forbidden until the twelfth century—and it has a restful plainness. I am an Anglican and find Roman Catholic decoration fussy. At Sénanque Abbey there is nothing but limestone—no frescoes, no treasures. It is built to express order and above all light.

Saint Bernard said: "Night will be engulfed in the victory of dawn, shadow and darkness shall disappear, and the splendor of the true Light shall invade the whole space: above, below, within, for in the morning we are already filled with His mercy."

The history of monasticism is resonant in this place. It was ransacked in the sixteenth century by Protestant Huguenots during the Wars of Religion. It wasn't until King Henry of Navarre issued the Edict of Nantes in 1598 that the wars came to an end.

I am reminded of this during the car journey, watching the news on my iPhone that Nantes Cathedral is in flames. I hope it will not be another Notre-Dame. There is something about the destruction of cathedrals that inspires awe and terror, just as the ruins of monasteries evoke thoughtfulness and melancholy.

By the nineteenth century, a new community of Cistercian monks named the Monks of the Immaculate Conception had moved in and started to make a living by growing lavender and keeping bees. Not much has changed since then. This is not a vocation taken lightly. Probationary training takes five years, then a further two years as a novice and three years of temporary commitment. Only then does a monk take his vows.

It is a kind of transfiguration into a world utterly unlike our own. It is without appetite or ambition or society; I was going to say without love but that is because I could not comprehend the idea of loving humanity in general rather than in particular. The Cistercians might say they love humankind through Jesus.

It is a lovely route to Gordes, past fields of sunflowers and avenues of limes—said to have been planted to provide shade for Napoleon's marching armies. We pass through Apt, where we have in the past watched the Tour de France come through the wide streets, cheered by lines of spectators. My husband and I sent our cycling-mad student daughter to buy beers while we were waiting, and in those minutes she missed the whizzing parade of cyclists. We have all learned patience since. I am aware that memories of family deeply bond my husband and me and I am afraid of the terrible loneliness of the monks.

There is no Tour de France during the COVID pandemic, but there are individual cyclists, with calf muscles like boulders, as they toil up and down these hills.

We pass the vineyards and fields of corn under the sky, the primary colors of a David Hockney. The satnav on the minibus-size rental car we are driving is taking us along narrow back roads, then up the almost vertical road leading to the fortress city of Gordes, scattering the walkers, down the other side of the hill, round countless bends and there below in a valley, on a carpet of lavender, are the pencil-colored Romanesque curves and slate roofs of the abbey. It is a ravishing setting. There is nothing forbidding about the building. It looks like a sanctuary.

I have only five minutes until admission ends at 11:00 A.M. for the day of prayers. I grab my pillow, sheets, and towels.

Sheets and towels were listed in the instructions that I was sent by the abbey, but I have also brought an extra pillow. I know this is a long way from the teachings of Saint Bernard of Clairvaux.

I hurry to the front section of the abbey, which is open to the public, and at the shop—selling beeswax and postcards—I ask the way to the community of monks. A bell is ringing as I dash with my trailing sheets around the hillside to the private monastery. I pass some scouts digging the path, run down courtyard steps, shout for directions, and I'm in the door with one minute to go. I stand panting and remorseful with my bulging bags like Maria from *The Sound of Music*.

Inside, the reception area resembles an empty disaster-zone health clinic. There is a waiting room with miscellaneous chairs and a picture of a saint whom I recognize as Saint Bernard. He would appreciate the modesty of the surroundings.

Opposite the waiting room is a row of hooks, for monastic dress, and behind it a picture of the Dome of the Rock in Jerusalem. I am reminded that monks and soldiers were of the same cloth in medieval times, and that the Crusades were part of the foundation of monasticism. Universities and hospitals grew out of monasticism, but that does not mean the origins were peaceful.

I hum under my breath the hymn now considered too bellicose for many church services but still used by the Salvation Army:

Onward Christian soldiers,
marching as to war,
With the cross of Jesus,
going on before!

Then I remember that I must not make any noise. I stand at the empty reception desk wondering what to do. There is a sign that reads: Merci de Bien Vouloir Respecter Le Silence Ici.

I don't want to call out and there is no bell on the reception desk, just a bottle of hand sanitizer. Behind the desk are a couple of chairs, and on the wall a picture of Jesus. I guiltily bend down to my bag to fish out my phone. As I scrabble around, I retrieve two phones, my own and my husband's. Neither has reception. My sense of monastic peace is broken by the realization that my husband is going to kill me when he realizes that I have his phone and I am incommunicado. It had been ceaselessly beeping all morning with messages about a crucial business Zoom meeting taking place the next day.

At that moment a door opens and a monk appears in his white gown and dark tunic. He has a long snowy beard and a high forehead and he goes by the name of Frère Hôtelier because he greets the guests. He is puzzled by the amount of bedding I have brought, indicating that there is no need for it.

The Cistercians speak as little as possible and my French is schoolgirl standard so we converse only as necessary. He shows me my room, a narrow wooden bed with a thin sheet and cover. There is a table, and a basin behind a yellowish cupboard. The shared lavatories and showers are on the floor above. So far, so boarding school. I gratefully swap the flat pillow for my bouncier one.

I look out from the window at the smooth stone frontage of the church. It is peaceful but not silent. There is scaffolding across the building and you can hear the hammer and chisel of the workers, although there is none of the banter you might expect to go with a group of male workmen. The builders, like the scouts, do not talk. Even the birds here seem silent, but that is partly because it is midday and midsummer.

On my desk is a laminated itinerary for the day. This is a place of routine.

I have become used to the fixed days of my grandson. Wake at 6:30 A.M., bottle, breakfast, bed, play, lunch, bottle, bed, play, supper, bottle, bed.

My own routine is usually iPhone led. My screen time is about eleven hours a day during lockdown and my head feels like a bees' nest.

The routine of the abbey is this:

04:30 Vigiles
07:45 Laudes
11:45 Messe
18:00 Vêpres suivies de l'adoration du Saint Sacrement
20:15 Complies

Prayer, reflection, and labor. All in silence.

The first prayers I get to is Mass. In order to reach the chapel, I go through a succession of heavy wooden doors into stone anterooms and then I reach the cloisters. They are graceful and pristine, fairly recently restored—flagstones, carved limestone pillars through which you glimpse a symmetrical inner garden of roses, rosemary, and hydrangeas, arranged within squares of box hedge and a pool of clear water at the center.

There is an alcove with a delicate stone statue of Mary and Jesus, carved with the same mystical serenity that I remember from the Black Madonna of Montserrat. At one side of the cloister is the beautiful barrel-vaulted chapter house.

A glimpse of a white robe moving across the other side; monks may come here for private prayer, Lectio Divina, but they should not be spoken to. I feel as if I have witnessed a unicorn or a ghost.

The tranquility of the cloister is part of the architecture of silence. The great arches represent the divine world, the smaller arches the human dimensions. The square of the cloister nestles under the right hand of the cross, represented by the church.

According to the abbey guidebook, twelve small paired columns represent the tribes of Israel. It is an image of Jerusalem; "Hail, holy land! Land of human sorrows and divine mercies."

The cloister is described in my book as a representation from the Song of Songs. This is my favorite book in the Bible, a sensuous depiction of an Eden and of a great love. It can be read as passionate dialogue between King Solomon and the Queen of Sheba, or as an allegory of the soul's quest for union with God. "Your breasts are like two fawns, like twin fawns of a gazelle that browse among the lilies." The meaning of this mystical book has been much studied over the centuries. The Venerable Bede, who loved the Song of Songs and recited verses from it in his austere cell, saw the bridegroom as Jesus Christ and the bride as the Catholic Church.

In the coolness of the cloisters I remember these lines from the book: "Flowers appear on the earth; the season of singing has come, the cooing of doves is heard in our land."

The season of singing has not come in the world of lockdown. There is no music in the churches. There is a cruel epidemiological twist to COVID, which is that it has silenced the sublime. Choirs cannot sing for fear of shedding droplets; there has been no *St. Matthew Passion* at Easter and it looks as if we will not have Handel's *Messiah* at Christmas.

However, the monks in this abbey have continued to sing psalms, a cappella, every single day through the lockdown.

I push at a heavy oak door that leads to the chapel. It is larger and emptier than I expected, with a wide vaulted ceiling and limestone floor. At the far end is a stone altar, with two candles on either side. Behind the altar, on an otherwise plain expanse of limestone wall, is a carving of Jesus on the cross and another of Mary.

There are chairs laid out, enough for about fifty people, but I sit on an oak bench at the back of the church, resting against the cool white stones. This monastery chapel has nothing extraneous. It is cool stone, bathed in light.

A line of monks enter, the younger ones appearing to glide up the central aisle, the older ones stiffer but still minimal in their movements. They take their seats in the altar pews and remain motionless for a few minutes. They have the profiles of an El Greco painting, the muted light catching their features.

Then the eldest lifts his head and strikes a note. Without expression, they follow it in choral harmony. The chubbiest-looking monk is also the bass, a ballast to the lighter tenor. There are no glances or smiles. They sing in somber humility.

The services of the day are fashioned around the hours of Good Friday and the spirit is of suffering rather than resurrection. A medieval chronicler wrote of the first Cistercians:

> *These holy monks wished to live unknown and forgotten in their deep solitude. Their austerities seemed beyond human endurance. They were half-naked—exposed to the most piercing cold of winter and the most burning heat of summer. To their continual labor they joined the most painful exercises: vigils, almost throughout the night, the divine office, spiritual lectures, long prayers. There was neither tumult, nor noise, nor confusion, nor complaint, nor dispute among them, nor intermission in their holy exercises.*

And yet the self-discipline is the route to peace of mind.

"The serenity of their faces," recorded William of Saint Thierry, "seemed the expression of the perfect peace which surrounds them in Heaven."

The melodic chanting of the psalms is alternated with readings. Nothing is hurried. The sound seems to come from the walls themselves but is contained within.

The snow-bearded frère then places a Communion vessel on the altar and swings incense around it. The other monks stand in front of him, one on each side, as exactly spaced as the candlesticks. Then they bow very low toward each other, creating a Renaissance tableau.

The senior monk prepares Communion wafers and lifts his eyes to the small congregation. We shuffle down the aisle, the students, pilgrims, and visitors, and then take our seats again. There are no further exchanges and the monks leave in silence except for one who remains seated. I have no impulse to leave either. I sit at the back, aware of his extraordinary stillness. I try to limit my natural movements. I do not cross or uncross my legs. I look only at the altar. The longer I am still, the more natural it becomes. I am not even aware of my breathing. It is a stillness that I can only describe as peace.

I have missed the bell for lunch but find the dining room, which looks out to the garden and the neat rows of vegetable allotments. There are about six tables and a few guests already eating at their laid places. I take a red-checked napkin from my pigeonhole and sit down next to a lone man in his sixties. I find out no more about him, not his nationality nor his family nor his interests. We eat in silence.

My neighbor does smile, however, and he passes me the steel tray of cold French beans, sardines, cheese, bread, and peaches. Out of a small speaker comes piped harpsichord. Without conversation, I eat more quickly, and after looking about the room, I pull back my chair and take my plate and cutlery to the small kitchen. I wash them up, put them on the rack, and then head back to my room.

I take the chair to the window and try to recreate my pose in the chapel. I will just sit here and look out of the window at the courtyard. But stillness cannot be summoned. I cannot look outdoors without wanting to go into the sunshine.

In the full heat of a South of France midday sun, I shut the front door, my room key in my pocket, and skip back round to the front of the abbey.

I am in the world again. Here are families and couples arm in arm, calling, chattering, laughing, posing, and taking selfies. Everything seems louder than it did before. Lockdown restrictions have only recently been lifted and this is a chance for everyone to head for the lavender fields and enjoy being outdoors. It seems as if the whole of Avignon has descended on this valley.

I walk up the hill at the front of the abbey. At the top of the path, in the midst of the dappled sunlight of trees, is a wooden cross and a celestial view of the abbey nestling in the valley. I wander further up through the lavender fields, the cabbage-white butterflies flitting between the rows—my husband's phone in my pocket pings angrily with unanswered messages. I walk briskly down the path again until I reach no service.

On the other side of the abbey, past the neatly laid-out vegetable crops, is rocky woodland. The trees here are thorny, the path blocked from time to time by small landslides of slate and limestone. It feels like a pilgrim's path, dusty and sharp with stones, so I persevere. One little track becomes a tributary of another. The sun is unforgivingly hot and flies are stinging my burning arms. But there are also powder-blue scabious meadow flowers and velvety brown moths. Saint Bernard wrote, "Woods and rocks will teach you what no other master can."

It was here that Petrarch, the Italian Renaissance poet and scholar, is said to have walked, during a tour of the region. Petrarch also climbed nearby Mount Ventoux. But he had a revelation that he should concentrate on the inner life rather than even on the beauty of nature.

I turned my inward eye upon myself and from that time not a syllable fell from my lips until we reached the bottom again. We look about us for what is to be found only within.

I am now on the wrong side of the monastery and cannot find a track to take me back. There is a small path, with a sign of a walker and a red line through it. I follow it back to the abbey but there is a deep ditch and a wall that I cannot vault over to get back to the vegetable garden. A scout appears from nowhere and leads me to a door, which opens into the monastery shop.

Hot and flustered and bitten, I am back in time for vespers. The handful of monks are in the choir stalls, in a fraternity of silence, waiting for the note. Most are gray haired and bearded. Their strength is invisible.

It could be a scene from the French film *Of Gods and Men*, based on the true story of a group of Cistercian Trappist monks who lived and worked among the Muslim population of Algeria in the 1990s.

As the Islamic militia grew more threatening, they chose to stay in their monastery rather than leave the country. They were waiting for their courage and faith to be tested. They were taken hostage at Christmas and the final scene of the film is of them trudging in deep snow to their beheading.

The prayer and rhythm of the monastery is captured in detail in the film, for it is an explanation for their fortitude at the end. The abbot, Christian de Chergé, left a testimony behind.

> *I could not desire such a death; it seems to me important to state this; How could I rejoice if the Algerian people I love were indiscriminately accused of my murder? My death, obviously, will appear to confirm those who hastily judged me naive or idealistic: "Let him tell us now what he thinks of it!"*
>
> *But they should know that . . . for this life lost, I give thanks to God. In this "thank you" which is said for everything in my life from now on, I certainly include you, my last minute friend who will not have known what you are doing. . . . I commend you to the God in whose face I see yours. And may we find each other, happy "good thieves" in Paradise, if it please God, the Father of us both.*

I watched *Of Gods and Men* on a winter's afternoon in Norfolk because a great Dominican friar and priest, named Timothy Radcliffe, told me that it contained the answer to my questions about truth and silence. In Radcliffe's book, *Alive in God: A Christian Imagination*, he asks if we have lost the sense of the transcendent. For all our connectivity and information, we find it hard to grasp meaning.

The motto of the Dominican order is *Veritas* (truth). The thirteenth-century Dominican friar, Saint Thomas Aquinas, drew upon pagan philosophers and Islamic teaching as sources of truth. He believed in a community of truth: that truth is beauty and beauty is truth.

When I asked Timothy Radcliffe, in his study piled with books, if he had found truth, he told me: "I believe there are truths but I don't know what they mean. I believe that God is good, but what does that mean?"

This seems to me the appeal of the cloisters at Sénanque. You can experience silence and truth even if you cannot rationalize or explain it. And I think I recognize in the monks what Radcliffe calls "the intimacy of silence with fellow brethren." The loneliness of the monks' lives is not loneliness at all. And their vows of poverty, chastity, and obedience are not confining but liberating.

One of the monks, a tall man with a smooth Roman head and deep-set eyes, moves to stand in front of the altar, ramrod-straight for about twenty minutes. Another kneels.

Then the senior frère returns, assuming an outer robe of ceremonial white and a hood. He moves to a lamp-lit decorated ark with a spire and a cross. He takes out a small object made of gold and glass, holds it up, and places it on the altar. It shines like a mirror.

The monks and the pilgrims look at it; we are completely still and the chapel is silent. Early-evening light pours through the stone window nearest to the altar. The tiniest rustle feels vexatious. This is a silence that floods through you like oxygen. It is what peace feels like.

After more than half an hour of stillness, the monks move as if out of a trance. I start. It is as if statues have come to life. I cross myself and drop a knee, which has become a habit. Then suddenly brisk, we make our way out of the chapel. I realize my vocal chords are becoming rusty with lack of use and I have started to look upward to avoid eye contact.

So when the Frère Hôtelier approaches me at the door of the refectory and asks me in English if I am well, I am surprised and pleased. Is this a sort of spiritual happy hour when we can exchange the pleasantries and banalities that I am used to outside the abbey?

He smiles gently and says he would like to ask something of me. Would I stay to the end of the meal this time rather than leaving the table once I have finished eating?

"We are a group," he says. "It is more convivial."

I had misread the community of silence. I thought that silence was the absence of a relationship, but in fact it was the opposite. I sit resolutely through a supper consisting of an avocado, a tomato, a leaf of lettuce, and heavily boiled zucchini and carrots, accompanied by piped music from "Greensleeves." Someone pushes back their chair, but it is only to fetch bread for the tables. We wait for the last person in the room to finish their final carrot. I note it but am careful not to react. And then everyone rises as one and assumes a line into the kitchen, where plates are handed from one person to the next to be washed and dried. Imagine a family Christmas day of washing up. But all done in silence.

I return to my room and realize *with excitement* that it is only fifteen minutes to evening prayers, called *complies*. The evening sun illuminates the east cloister—it creates white tombs of light across the flagstones. I rest by a stone pillar, looking across the garden square, up at the darkening stone of the chapel and the evening sky above it. It resembles ink on papyrus, shades of violet blue and dove gray on muslin weave. Swifts over the abbey are the only creatures that move on this quiet evening.

I slip into the back of the chapel, bow, cross myself, and sit on my oak bench. The monks take their places at the altar pews. Since I cannot follow closely the language or the liturgy I am content to absorb the Gregorian chants and even more the silences in between. The service is ancient, serious, penitent. There are no platitudes here, no topicality.

I am used to the megaphone of current affairs and the jumpiness of a pandemic. Here, these rumbling bass voices mingling with the tenors produce harmony both ancient and present. It is the sound of eternity. The monks are old enough to fear the effects of COVID but what should they fear, when they are poised between two worlds?

At the end of the service, the snow-bearded monk holds up a leafy branch and gently waves it above the heads of the other monks and, as he walks down the aisle, the heads of our little congregation of visitors.

The lights of the chapel are switched off, but once again I am rooted to my bench. I, who have never been able to sit through meetings and have a shockingly short concentration span, want nothing more than this. Sitting in shadows and stillness, looking at a limestone wall, and the wooden image of the cross. Simplicity and silence.

My bedroom has also become dear to me. There is a breeze through the long open window and I look out at the wooded hillside and the stone. I have never known such concentrated stillness. I look up at Venus and then bow my head, the gesture that has already become natural.

And the hard, narrow bed beckons an unbroken sleep. For one day at least, the sleep of the innocent.

The bell in the tower sounds at 4:15 A.M. for vigiles. I wonder if I can sleep through it. Surely I can miss one daily service out of seven?

But each one is subtly different because they are fixed to the holy calendar. I slip on a dress, brush my teeth, and comb my hair. This all feels odd since it was not that long ago that I was taking off my dress and brushing my teeth for bed. This is not night, nor day. It feels like a fire alarm, or a flight.

In the darkness, I feel my way down the steps, then along the familiar route, past two wooden doors, into the cloister and toward the chapel. There are only four monks and only three in the congregation. Even the monks yawn a little and wipe their glasses.

Yet the first sung note brings concentration and with it gladness. The predawn hours of a news program are coffee and adrenaline. Here they are contemplation. The lack of coffee and indeed of alcohol the night before already brings a quietness of mind. The lack of sleep encourages a spiritual alertness. I have never felt this equilibrium before. Attentive and yet still.

The service finishes at about 5:30 A.M. and I wonder about going back to bed. But dawn is rising and the rocks and woodland are becoming three-dimensional. I take the Saint Bernard route up the stony path I followed yesterday, and at the top of the hilly ridge, I watch the sun come up. A single cloud in the shape of a chariot is lit orange and yellow.

Below me, I see light curling across the slate roof of the monastery.

I make my way down the path and up the empty road on the other side, which will soon be full of tourists. I want to see the lavender fields, lit by morning sun. At the edge of a lavender field, I watch a black-and-navy butterfly, spotted with white, on sunlit oak leaves. Solitude becomes one with nature. I sit on a stone by a tree cloaked in lichen, and assume the pose of the chapel. Head bowed, hands together, completely still.

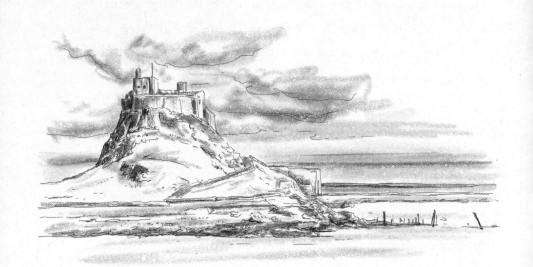

Chapter 8

LIVING ON
THE EDGE
LINDISFARNE

T he Venerable Bede said of Saint Cuthbert: "He pre-
ferred the monastery to the world."

The desert fathers chose barren places under piti-
less sun; the Celts chose the wildest shores. Their Irish monasteries were stations of penitence—rocky outposts, lashed by
waves, insulated from Rome by their own folklore and geography. Celtic monasticism is woven into the history of local kings,
poets, druids, and spirits.

An island that has long fascinated me is Skellig Michael,
west of Kerry. Its twin peaks, thrusting from the swell of the
Atlantic Ocean, are now home to puffins and cormorants, but
once housed a sixth-century monastic settlement. Stone was
quarried to create drystone hive cells, reached by dramatic, vertiginous steps. There was no fresh water, little access or means of
escape, but there was prayer and the moods of the Atlantic for
spiritual sustenance. The monks carved a hundred stone crosses
on the little island; this was the rock of Christianity.

Penitence was not just the treatment, it was the cure. It was monks medicine. Columbanus, one of the sixth-century founding fathers of Irish monasticism, wrote: "For the doctors of the body also compound their medicines in diverse kinds; thus they heal wounds in one manner, sickness in another ... so also should spiritual doctors treat with diverse kinds of cures the wounds of the soul." In the sixteenth century, the island was known across Christendom as a merciless penitential station, and for pilgrims it was the hardest destination.

In the nineteenth century, long after the last monks had abandoned the island, Lord Dunraven produced the first archaeological plans of Skellig Michael. "The scene," he wrote, "is one so solemn and so sad that none should enter here but the pilgrim and the penitent. The sense of solitude, the vast heaven above and the sublime monotonous motion of the sea beneath would oppress the spirit, were not the spirit brought into harmony."

Alas, it defeats me before I even get there. I book the bed-and-breakfast and the boat before lockdown, taking precise advice on seasons and tides. Flights to Ireland are secured, the ferry is plan B. Then the Irish government closes the island and slaps a quarantine rule on all arrivals to Kerry. I grumble to an Irish journalist friend, who says rules are not exactly rules in Ireland—except where monks are concerned.

No boat owner would defy the government, even though they are broke and the trip is into open sea, which would disperse COVID droplets like sea spray. Spiritual heritage matters more than economy.

Celtic monasticism records three great landmarks: Skellig Michael, Iona in Scotland, and Lindisfarne on the coast of Northumberland, in the northeast of England.

The edge of existence has a visionary quality. Between land and sea, between reality and imagination, between heaven and earth. Iona Abbey, just off the Isle of Mull, on the west coast of Scotland, was where Christianity crossed from Ireland to the mainland. The Irish monk Saint Columba, or Columcille, left Ireland in AD 565, with twelve companions, and landed on Iona.

Iona, it turns out, is also closed for the duration of the pandemic. When Columcille died there in AD 697 he caused a ferocious storm lasting for three days, so no outsiders could attend his burial. The spell of austerity and unworldliness was not to be broken.

A similar spell falls on the summer of 2020—I cannot reach Iona for all my pleading and many online bookings.

How to be a pilgrim? I turn to the third center of monasticism, which is Lindisfarne, or to use its other name, Holy Island, the three-mile thread of rock and grass, cut adrift by tides, near the border with Scotland. I can follow in the footsteps of Saint Aidan, the seventh-century Irish monk who traveled first to Iona and then on to Lindisfarne, bringing Christianity to Northumbria. Some believe Aidan should be a unifying saint for the United Kingdom.

Lindisfarne also inspired the eighth-century monk the Venerable Bede, who spent his life in Northumberland at the monastery of Jarrow and died there in 735.

Bede loved stories of Britain. His great work, *Historia Ecclesiastica*, shows how the imagination can transport; his took him far beyond the walls of the monastery of Jarrow. He described Britain, for instance, in these terms:

An island rich in crops and trees . . . remarkable too for its rivers, which abound with fish, especially salmon and eels, and for copious springs. Seals as well as dolphins are frequently captured and even whales, besides these are various shellfish among which are mussels and enclosed in these are often found pearls of every color, red and purple, violet and green, but mostly white.

His was a blend of observation and poetic reverie.

Saint Cuthbert owes his fame to the writing of Bede. Cuthbert grew up across the border in Scotland and became a monk after a vision on the night of the death of Saint Aidan. Pilgrims still walk Saint Cuthbert's Way, from Melrose to Saint Boswells, Jedburgh, Morebattle, Kirk Yetholm, Wooler, Fenwick, and finally Lindisfarne, where they cross at low tide, navigating their course and the rising water by the pathway of poles anchored in the sand. In AD 684, Cuthbert became bishop of Lindisfarne, but sought further solitude on a rock at the edge of the island. As Bede wrote, he went as far as he could to "stand vigil in the icy water."

Cuthbert's body was removed from Lindisfarne following Viking raids in the ninth century and later taken to Durham. When his tomb was opened in September 1104, a pocket Gospel, dated AD 710, was discovered inside the coffin. A thirteenth-century note explains: "The Gospel of Saint John . . . was found at the head of our blessed father Cuthbert lying in his tomb in the year of his translation."

Literature is a magnificent legacy of monasticism. It was the monks who copied out books that might otherwise have been lost, and they did so in writing so exquisite that it became an art form. The Lindisfarne Gospels are a sublime example of monastic illuminated manuscripts. History records that they were the labor of Eadfrith, a bishop on Holy Island in the eighth century. In the tenth century, a footnote was added by a Northumberland priest named Aldred:

> *Eadfrith bishop of the Church of Lindisfarne,*
> *He, in the beginning, wrote this book for God and*
> *Saint Cuthbert and generally for all the holy folk*
> *Who are on the island.*
> *And Æthilwald bishop of the Lindisfarne-islanders,*
> *bound and covered it without, as he knew well how to do.*
> *And Billfrith the anchorite, he forged the*
> *ornaments which are on the outside and*
> *bedecked it with gold and with gems and*
> *also with gilded silver-pure wealth.*

I have a friend named Eyob Derillo, who works on illuminated manuscripts at the British Library. Surely, he must have come across the Gospels? I would give anything to see them. Eyob replies that he too would love to look at them, but the rooms are closed at the moment and anyway they are only on display for certain periods. They are too precious and rare to be exposed to the light. We must ration ourselves on delight.

I write to Eyob's head of department, who puts me on to Dr. Claire Breay, head of Ancient Medieval and Early Modern Manuscripts. May I come to see the Lindisfarne Gospels? She replies with crisp precision:

> *The Lindisfarne Gospels are displayed according to a schedule agreed [sic] by the British Library board in 2009 which means they are on display for eighteen months in every twenty-four and rested off-display in secure storage for six months from April to September in each even-numbered year. With any luck, they will be back in the Library's Treasures Gallery from October 2020.*

In London, the museums start to reopen in August, one by one, and I watch intently the plans for the British Library. The announcement finally comes: It is reopening on July 22.

I am back on to Dr. Breay like a seabird. Is it time? Can I come? She responds again with patient scrupulousness: The Lindisfarne Gospels are not on display at the moment, but I will be able to see them in the Treasures Gallery from next month; I can, however, see a very high-quality facsimile in the Manuscripts Reading Room, which is now open.

But it is the original I want to see, not a facsimile. The great qualities that I have to learn from monasticism are diligence and patience.

I must wait to see the Gospels, but I can go to Holy Island, where they came from, and I can follow the trail of Cuthbert and Bede in Northumberland. Bede is easy to find, because he did not travel. He was a child oblate at Jarrow, a pupil of Abbot Ceolfrid, founder of Jarrow monastery.

We equate our physical confinement during the pandemic with diminished lives, but Bede shows that our imagination is limitless. His love of knowledge was monastic—it was an end in itself. He believed that all knowledge is connected, which is perhaps why he was so taken with the Song of Songs in the Bible. It is poetic, allegorical, mystical. Bede linked religion and evidence-based science with an intellectual suppleness. He understood layered meaning.

During a warm August week, when the British people are weighing up risk against freedom and starting to travel, my husband and I throw a case into the car and head off for the great northern city of Durham and then Lindisfarne. In other words, we are following in the steps of the Venerable Bede and Saint Cuthbert, but with the promise of bed and breakfasts rather than sore feet.

You can walk the boundaries of Bede's existence; you can stand on the patch of grass, marked out by stones, next to the twelfth-century church, which was his cell from the age of seven. Jarrow is deserted when we get there and Saint Paul's Church is locked. A sign says that all church services are canceled until further notice. But it is not hard to imagine how, in the seventh and eighth centuries, this patch of earth grew to be one of Europe's most influential centers of learning and culture. The swans flap their wings on the Don River at the bottom of the grassy bank; the river flows into the Tyne and on to the North Sea, and in the distance are the cranes of Jarrow's nearby port.

Bede dreamed of Egypt and Arabia and was in sight of trade and travel by river and sea.

Bede and Cuthbert are united in Durham Cathedral, built to house the latter's remains. As we get there, the weather is darkening over the forbidding stone squatting aloft the city. The cathedral, described by Sir Walter Scott as "half church of God, half castle against the Scots," is a rebuke to the sunny, frivolous South that we have left behind.

When Cuthbert died on the hermetic island of Inner Farne, within sight of Lindisfarne, torches were lit to proclaim his death. In AD 995, his relics were brought to Durham. Cuthbert is the North's proudest saint, the towering figure of Celtic monasticism, and you feel his presence in the stern beauty of Durham. Normally, visitors enter the cathedral via the Norman nave, stopping in front of the great wooden door and its sanctuary knocker. But during COVID, we wind our way into the Galilee Chapel on the west. Families in anoraks, denied other forms of leisure, gaze up instead at the great walls.

Behind the hand sanitizer station and the contact-tracing book is the shrine of the Venerable Bede. The smooth plain slab on a stone base, surrounded by four candles, is easily missed if you are not looking for it. It has an aura of modesty, yet a profound authority. Bede's prayer is copied out beside it: "Grant me one day to come to you, the fountain of all wisdom and to stand forever before your face." A small descriptive plaque nearby calls the Venerable Bede the greatest scholar of his age and the father of English history. The mother of a small child looking the other way, sighs, "I love Bede." Her daughter drags her away.

Cuthbert's shrine is closed but I stand still in the nave, as I have learned from the Cistercians, staring ahead at the high altar and the rose window where the monks would have prayed and where, pre-COVID, the cathedral choir would have been singing in the carved wooden stalls, before the marble sanctuary floor. A cathedral built for a monk.

We drive on up the coast road. The sky clears above curving hills of sheep, stone walls, and copses. All is green and soft. A light rain falls and the air is sweet. We walk to Bamburgh Castle, another daunting fortress on a hill, but this time built in red sandstone. Below is a village cricket ground; the field must have the best setting in the country. It is evening and the colors of the sky above the castle are a combination of bright white and deep gray. Light beams down as if through prison bars. The wet sand forms patterns on a path of light. The castle is a silhouette and the lighthouses flash from the Farne Islands. No wonder Turner painted here. I cast my mind further back to the stealthy Viking raids and the shapes of the monks gazing out to sea.

I look across to Lindisfarne, a strip of land, as if sketched in pencil, with a hump that in daylight would show itself as the fortress castle. Above the pencil line is a second line, illuminated. It is a halo of light across Lindisfarne. We walk over the dunes down to the harbor. The light is now violet ink, the sky low over the waveless sea. We eat fish and chips by the sea wall, watched beadily by the gulls, and gaze at the Farne Islands. A small blinking vessel is returning safely to the harbor, leaving behind the dark isolation of Cuthbert's island. The Romans called Lindisfarne *Insula Medicata*—island where balm was made.

The gauzy morning mist lifts over the hillside pastures of sheep and the line of evergreen trees above. I think of Bach's aria "Sheep May Safely Graze." I watch the flock, content beneath a cloudless sky, the air waterfall fresh. We drive down to the coastal causeway, which is open, and over the sea-wet road to Holy Island. It is busy with day-trippers and pilgrims. The parking lot is almost full by 9:30 A.M. and walkers are heading in small groups, familiar since COVID, to the sights of the twelfth-century Lindisfarne Priory, the castle, and the pubs. It is in the early days of face masks and we grimace with embarrassment as we put them on. Mask on for the museum, mask off for outside.

I am looking for Mark Douglas, who works for English Heritage. He waves at us from the entrance, stout, with hair like barn owl feathers and Viking-blue eyes. Saint Aidan used Lindisfarne as a base to convert heathens to a Christian God, and Mark Douglas uses it to convert us to his passion for medieval monasteries. "Just don't get me going on chantry chapels," he says, his face alight with pleasure. His accent is Hartlepool. Mark was a sheet metal welder until, in his late twenties, he developed a profound interest in Anglo-Saxon churches. He went to Durham University to study churches and then medieval archaeology, and after ten years came away with a PhD in the subject.

His wife, who had been his childhood sweetheart, would sit patiently outside in the car as he looked at arches and windows. Her favorite place was Rievaulx Abbey in Yorkshire because she could sit on a bench looking down at the valley. He would stop what he was doing from time to time and see her figure, on the bench, happily reading. Mark says he still feels a tingle down his spine at Rievaulx. When his wife died two years ago, he missed her very much. His children, wanting to console their father, came up with a trip of a lifetime. They took him to Constantinople, as he calls it (now Istanbul), to look at the Sophia church (now mosque).

A pilgrimage of medieval monasticism.

Northumberland had held stubbornly to Celtic monasticism but the monks of Lindisfarne became enamored by books and learning and therefore European civilization. This led them back to Rome. The tension must be in the soil. The Northeast was where the swell of the Brexit vote originated.

Mark shows us the pillars and window in the Romanesque style of Durham, with high rainbow arches, but here looking out to a desolate sea. He is most expansive standing in the spot of what was once the infirmary where the monks were bled. Monks understood pandemics. They lived through centuries of plagues. In AD 541, the Plague of Justinian, named for the Roman emperor in Constantinople, spread across the Near East and Europe, killing about twenty-five million people. There was another great plague in the middle of the seventh century, of which Bede wrote: "The pestilence came."

Mark, like Cuthbert and Aidan, loves Lindisfarne above all for its extremity. He has been to Iona and says that Skellig, Iona, and Lindisfarne all share the same spirit.

For the next few days, I make my peace with that spirit. Our hotel room backs onto the grounds of the ruined priory; my window looks out at the statue of Saint Aidan and the Celtic cross. Beyond the priory is the heugh, a strip of land next to a precipice used as a lookout. It was from here that the monks rowed out in their small boats for Jarrow.

I watch, from the west-facing window, the castle on the rock turn rose in the sunset, then darken by degrees, as the sky becomes a kaleidoscope of colors. We walk up to the heugh to look down at the cross of Cuthbert. Across the water are some sand flats, between Lindisfarne and Bamburgh, and from them comes an unearthly moaning. I raise my binoculars to see the source of the sound. It is a colony of seals, writhing and flipping across each other, in search of a place to rest for the night.

In the early morning, as we rise at 6:00 A.M. for a walk, the same noise carries across the island. I walk past the boat repair yard, with its coils of rope and oyster nets. A woman with a complicated camera and pink hair nods at me, and then says in an American accent : "What *is* that noise?" She is watching my face as if to take her lead from my expression. "It is the seals, singing," I say, and we both smile.

Cuthbert was drawn to the sea, as Bede, who loved him, described:

> That man of God, approaching the sea with mind made resolute, went into the waves up to his loincloth; and once he was soaked as far as his armpits by the tumultuous and stormy sea. Then coming up out of the sea, he prayed, bending his knees on the sandy part of the shore, and immediately there followed in his footsteps two little sea animals, humbly prostrating themselves on the earth; and licking his feet, they rolled upon them, wiping them with their skins and warming them with their breath. [Otters.]

Cuthbert also protected the nests on Inner Farne and let the eider ducks, known as Cuddy's ducks, into the chapel.

Alone with the gulls we walk around the island, on paths that disappear into seagrass, or meet marsh and dune, until we come to the posts forming a straight line in the sand across the causeway to the mainland. They were submerged last night but now a pilgrims' path is emerging. By the time we leave the island at 9:00 A.M. the water has retreated from the road and cars of day-trippers are bumper to bumper. The end of the world is accessible again.

Winter trudges in, the rain comes in sheets, and the prime minister warns of a second wave of COVID. North West and North East England are badly hit. I am settled in London for my final month at the BBC, trying to keep an office open. An email arrives from Claire Breay at the British Library: "Many apologies for not getting back to you sooner. I wanted to let you know that the Lindisfarne Gospels will be back on display in the Treasures Gallery this week. Because of the COVID restrictions, if you would like to come to see it on display, you would currently need to book a slot."

I am on my laptop faster than for Christmas Waitrose deliveries. I have a slot. It is 1:00 P.M. and I need to be there fifteen minutes early. On the day appointed, I am still on a corporate Zoom call at 12:30. There is nothing else for it; I turn off audio and video, plead a lost connection, and run for the subway. I am at the British Library entrance at 1:05, in the cascading rain, one of a handful of people with rain hoods, steamed glasses, and brandished phones. Mine is scanned, and my heart skips as I walk toward the entrance of the Treasures Gallery. When

I started my monastery journey, I imagined desert, oceans, and distant lands. Now I am grateful for five stops on the subway and admission to a public building.

The gallery has cases of miscellaneous items, but I follow the floor arrows straight to the sacred texts. And there, eclipsing the rest in size and weight, are the Lindisfarne Gospels. It takes two people to carry them, and one to turn the page on display. I am told there is an added frisson when it is the turn of the first page of one of the Gospels, with its jeweled calligraphy.

The page on show at the moment is Saint Jerome's preface to the four Gospels, starting with the words *Plures Fuisse*—"there have been many." The letter *P* is a work of art, an animal head and uncoiled body in a loop and tail. Otherwise, the ink writing is notable for its extraordinary neatness. If the monks made a mistake, they would scratch out the letter and start again. Above the Latin text is an Old English translation, attributed to the tenth-century priest, Aldred. The curator, Kathleen Doyle, tells me later on the telephone that the English would have sounded more like German. I tell her I was struck by the tidiness of the scripts. They are ruled with a straight edge, sometimes with pricked holes to ensure the line. "Oh, calligraphers get so excited by that," she says warmly.

Next to the Lindisfarne Gospel is a relatively modest prayer book. This is the Gospel of Saint John, which lay in Cuthbert's coffin for four hundred years and still looks in gleaming condition. In the sepulchral darkness of the museum room in which silent figures follow signposted steps, wearing their plague masks, I think of the edge of the world where the Lindisfarne Gospels were transcribed and bound. Somehow a fusion of artistic

styles—the Celtic, the Germanic, and the Mediterranean—
were absorbed by the monks.

I ask Kathleen Doyle if there was something particular
about Lindisfarne that contributed to producing these Gospels.
She replies: "I went to Lindisfarne a couple of years ago to walk
across that causeway. I don't want to get too fanciful, but there is
a kind of luminosity about the place. The Gospels were a reflection of that interior spiritual life. They are a work of devotion."

When even a windswept island seemed not far enough, the
monks waded further into the waters. At Lindisfarne, geographical and spiritual extremity went hand in hand and out of them
came these incredible books. Desolation produced illumination.
Through the Gospels those monks conjured divine glory.

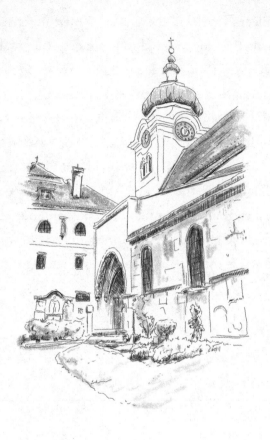

Chapter 9

MUSIC AND MONASTICISM

SALZBURG

Some listeners of the *Today* program during the heat of the election threatened to turn to the BBC's classical music channel Radio 3 and I cannot say that I blamed them. I made friends with one of Radio 3's most beauteous presenters, a violinist named Clemency Burton-Hill. She has large brown eyes and tumbling blond hair and is married to a handsome diplomat who used to be a royal official.

Clemency wrote a book called *Year of Wonder: Classical to Enjoy Day by Day*, and I asked her to choose a piece of music each month to cheer up the *Today* program. One day I came across her curled up fawn-like on a grubby office chair, looking out of the windows of New Broadcasting House. She said that she could not make headway at the BBC and was going to take a job at the classical radio station WQXR in New York.

A few months later, I heard terrible news. Clemency had suffered a massive brain hemorrhage and half her skull had been removed to release the pressure. During her seventeen-day coma, she believed that she saw "not really angels, but beings" who led her out of the darkness.

Her friends and family found a way of reviving her consciousness and memory. They played Bach, Brahms, Beethoven, and Handel. Clemency's friend, the violinist Nicola Benedetti, visited her months later and showed her how to play Bach's Partita in D Minor. "Music is the opposite of despair," Clemency told the BBC.

At the time that Clemency was learning to live again through music, I visited the Dominican friar Timothy Radcliffe in Oxford. He writes of the Christian imagination, by which he means that faith displays itself in many forms. The qualities of monasticism are reflected in music; in Beethoven and Bach, for instance.

Alfred Brendel said: "Silence is the basis of music. We find it before, after, in, underneath and behind the sound. Silence also ought to be the core of each concert." Monasticism and music are close.

Live music has been silenced during the pandemic. Churches closed, orchestras disbanded, cherubic choristers feared as transmitters of disease. My application for tickets to the Salzburg Festival at Easter is returned, canceled. Who can tell when we will hear music again?

It is Salzburg that leads the way, the first cuckoo of summer. The festival will go ahead as best it can in August. And I have tickets for Beethoven.

I am especially happy because it means that I can also see again the friend that I had made at the monastery in Egypt,

Professor Aho Shemunkasho, who teaches Aramaic at Salzburg University.

"What is your address?" I asked him on a Zoom call a month earlier. There is his smooth, earnest face, too close to the screen, surrounded by neat rows of books. He replies that he lives in the monastic district, just opposite Nonnberg Abbey. I repeat the name, because it has a familiar ring. He grins: "*Sound of Music.*"

A month later, the lady from the Salzburg tourist office asks when I phone to inquire about Nonnberg Abbey: "Is this about *The Sound of Music?*"

Salzburg is a musically serious city, which treats its heritage as the birthplace of Mozart as a defining honor. It has a Baroque cathedral with five organs. But for generations of Americans, Canadians, and British, Salzburg is basically Julie Andrews and "Do-Re-Mi."

I reply to the tourist lady that I am in fact coming to hear a Beethoven concert—and then I book a sing-a-long *Sound of Music* tour of the city. I say to my husband that I am musing on the title "Music and Monasticism" for this chapter.

"What about 'Nuns and Nazis'?" he suggests.

The film of the musical with Julie Andrews is almost as old as I am and yet it remains irresistible. The story, loosely based on the truth, is about a nun named Maria from the Benedictine Abbey of Nonnberg in Salzburg who comes to be governess to the seven children of the widowed Captain von Trapp. She falls in love with the naval hero, and the family flees Austria in 1938 rather than accept Nazi rule. The triumph of principle, patriotism, and prayer is unquestioned by Rodgers and Hammerstein.

I book flights to Salzburg, but all journeys are capricious as airlines weigh up whether it is commercially worth it, relative to the number of passengers. When the booking is canceled for the third time, we take the precaution of flying to Munich, close to the Austrian border, as students of *The Sound of Music* will know.

From Munich we board the train to Salzburg—choosing the quiet-zone carriage, although masks and cultural obedience mean all the carriages seem pretty quiet. On the other side of the aisle is a young ponytailed man, who flings down his ruck-sack and then sensitively lifts a violin case onto the overhead shelf.

From the window I watch the landscape change from arable to wide rivers and woods and finally the shapes of the eastern Alps and chalets with bright window boxes. We are crossing an invisible border into Austria.

It is hot and humid, spiked with a hint of mountain air, as the train stops in Salzburg. We have our COVID-free documents, but nobody asks for them because we have come through Munich. We are the only Brits here and may be the last for a while. A week later, the UK puts Austria on the quarantine list. But, for now, we seize the day.

We walk from the station past streets of chain cafés and discount shops to the old city. High up, dominating everything, is the castle, and tucked around the side of it, Nonnberg Abbey. I swing my hand luggage and declare that I have confidence in me.

We are booked in at a seminary, with views of a Capuchin monastery on a hill. It is a seventeenth-century Baroque building, next to Trinity Church, entered through a massive wooden door set within a stone arch on the main street. Above it a sign reads: Collegium Presbyterorum et Aluminorum.

Inside is a cool stone courtyard close to the cupola. Wide stone stairs on the left lead to the seminary; we are in guest rooms on the other side. The room is plain—a wardrobe, a chair and table, twin beds, a cross above the beds, a Bible on the bedside table. The tall window opens onto a side street of lively cafés and bars.

We wander around the streets, past the river in the late-afternoon sunshine, into Mozart Square and the cathedral. Bars, snack shops, and chocolate emporiums are all named after Mozart. Even the graffiti says Mozart.

And all around me I can hear the voice of Placido Domingo—I trace it to a recorded concert on a large screen in front of which are about ten rows of chairs. The audience is smiling nostalgically, remembering this fifteen-year-old performance, recalling the joyful liberation of lungs before COVID.

We walk on, past a shop dedicated to the English, selling cider and bric-a-brac. It is called Thatchers' and written on the blackboard in chalk is the one word: "Brexit." It is a single-minded representation of Britain. I want to add the name: Julie Andrews.

Then we find a steep road that rises above the rooftops of Salzburg. We can see the pale spires and domes of this religious city, and hear the bells and notes coming from churches and concert halls.

Do you remember the scene in *The Sound of Music* in which the children come to the abbey gates and beg the nuns to let them talk to Maria? Here is the hillside road that winds around the walls of the abbey. On the wall is a simple sign: Stiftskirche Nonnberg. And here is the whirly pale-gray wrought iron door, against which the children poked their faces to speak to the nuns. It is firmly locked now, as it was then, but I can see behind it a cobbled stone courtyard and a heavy oak door. There is something else that I recognize in the higher slope of the road leading up to a stone gateway.

It is where the von Trapps made their escape; the car is rolling down the hill. Film set meets sacred place. The folk of Salzburg maintain a studied ignorance of the film, yet Rodgers and Hammerstein brought crowds here. My professor, Aho, says that there was a scheme to turn his house into a *Sound of Music* elevator to save tourists the trouble of toiling up the steep road, but the nuns drew the line between entertainment and private prayer.

My husband and I eat a light supper of fish and salad in a side-street restaurant and then walk back to the peace of the seminary. It is quiet inside the room but also now swelteringly hot. We open the window wide. With its high ceiling and church-scale window, it is a room of remarkable acoustics. It is as if every table in the café has been relocated to our bedside. Conversations and laughter are trumpeted directly into my ear, even with the monastically thin pillow over my head. Then I notice, placed next to the Bible, a pack of earplugs.

Quiet eventually comes in the hour before dawn but this is also a country of early risers. At 5:00 A.M. there is an operatic bin collection below, which I first mistake for demolition of the building.

Yet downstairs, all is calm and orderly. Trainee priests sit murmuring at courtyard tables, patiently smoothing butter and jam onto their toast. The pale gray and white of the building is restful. I look up the hill at the monastery, established by the Capuchins, an order that arose in the sixteenth century to restore the Franciscan strictness. My merry-go-round night is fading in the scholarly light of day. Monasticism reasserts itself over deafening hedonism.

We walk along the river; then down heat-rising streets to pick up tickets for tonight's concert. There is music coming from the windows, from buskers, from hidden courtyards. I shuffle forward in Grandmother's footsteps in the six-foot-distanced queue and at last I have them in my hand—tickets for Beethoven's piano sonatas, once described as the New Testament to Bach's Old Testament.

We walk to the magnificent Salzburg Cathedral. The first cathedral, built by Bishop Virgil in AD 767, went up in flames more than once. Finally after yet another fire in the late sixteenth century, it was rebuilt by Archbishop Markus Sittikus as the first Baroque church north of the Alps. It dominates the center of Salzburg with its milky splendor.

En route is a shop and museum dedicated to *The Sound of Music*, sadly closed for the pandemic. There is a large sepia portrait of the real Maria von Trapp, more matronly and patient-looking than Julie Andrews. The Captain's portrait also lacks the matinee idol looks of Christopher Plummer, although it does radiate decency and determination.

The Sound of Music film crew wanted Salzburg Cathedral as the setting for Maria's wedding, the romantic aspiration for many thousands of girls, including me. When I was young, wedding dress dreams were a choice between Julie Andrews, Grace Kelly, or Princess Diana. I reckon Julie Andrews eclipsed the others. But Salzburg Cathedral turned down *The Sound of Music*, apparently in an act of high-minded musical disdain.

Let's face it, the cathedral does already have its own musical credentials. Mozart was baptized in the font and he composed sacred music here. As we proceed down the aisle—this is how Julie Andrews might have done it—we hear one of the smaller organs being played to the side of us. A young man with long pale hands repeats a refrain before quietly shuffling his sheets of music and disappearing. Is this how Mozart might have been glimpsed in the eighteenth century?

I remember Goethe's description of Mozart: "An inexplicable prodigy." Perhaps this is what Timothy Radcliffe meant when he talked about music being a route to faith. We cannot explain divinity but we know it when we encounter it.

In Mozart Square in the late afternoon, groups are strolling in the direction of the Mozart concert hall. They are dressed up, the women in bright silks with geometric patterns, in high heels and jewelry. They leave fragrant trails. I have become so unused to the sight of finery during lockdown that I gawk and follow them. We are all in search of music.

I am holding my tickets for Beethoven's piano sonatas played by the thirty-three-year-old Russian-born Berlin-based pianist Igor Levit. On Twitter, he describes himself as a human being. Citizen. Activist. Pianist. Critics might put pianist first. Like Mozart, Levit was playing the piano aged three, and later studied at the Mozarteum in Salzburg.

He is with the home crowd tonight. And they are milling outside, in joyous anticipation. The doors open and we make our way up the staircases, concertgoers in PPE. As the unassuming figure in loose black clothing appears onstage and sits before his piano, we are permitted to take off our masks, as if Beethoven might have mastery over the virus. The music transcends everything.

The sonatas tug at the thread of genius from Mozart to Beethoven. In 1792, an admirer wrote to the twenty-one-year-old Beethoven: "Through uninterrupted diligence you will receive Mozart's spirit from Haydn's hands."

Genius still requires the monastic virtue of labor. The Piano Sonata No. 2 in A Major combines the Baroque and the choral with a bit of thunder. Beethoven understood that music could reach beyond reason and express profound unspoken truths. The next sonata, No. 7 in D Major, is described as a "detailed study in melancholy."

The program notes say: "It is only the coda with its plunge into E flat minor and its ensuing chromatically rising bass line that gives us a true idea of the depths of the pain that have to be surmounted."

Music then an expression of suffering and of joy.

The solemn-looking pianist, wiping his damp fingers on his black cotton sleeves, returns for an encore, grins broadly, and plays some ragtime. Music must lift our spirits as well as expand our horizons.

The religiosity of Beethoven was not the same as that of Mozart. With Beethoven, it is more an expression of religious feeling than of dogma, while Mozart was more conventionally churchgoing. There is a deity in the two Beethoven masses, his Mass in C Major and *Missa Solemnis;* perhaps as he started to lose his hearing, his music took him into a new sphere.

The nineteenth-century musicologist Joseph d'Ortigue wrote: "Beethoven makes us hear angels' choirs, the organ's register, and the sounds of nature."

If I had to choose a musical route to monasticism, however, I would follow Mozart. Think of the heartbreaking choral sweetness of *Ave Verum Corpus*—composed for the feast of Corpus Christi, 1791, near the end of Mozart's life. Or the sacred simplicity of *Laudate Dominum*, composed in Salzburg, based on the psalm "Praise the Lord all ye nations." Or the unfinished Requiem Mass in D Minor. Mozart died in 1791, aged thirty-five.

Mozart composed Mass in C Major for the ordination of his friend Cajetan Hagenauer at Saint Peter's Abbey and this, along with his Requiem, is played every December 4 here, to mark his death.

Mozart's birthplace is a tall, canary-yellow townhouse on a main street in Salzburg, ground once owned by the Benedictine monks of Saint Peter's. The family of musicians rented the third floor from merchant landlords, and the rooms display their dedication to their art.

I look in wonder at Mozart's piccolo violin and harpsichord and the early editions of his music. Mozart's father, Leopold, was an accomplished musician who wrote a textbook on the violin. Picking up one of his son's childhood compositions—Mozart was writing piano concertos at the age of four—he shed tears over the imagination and mastery of the score. His son was a genius.

In the Mozart museum and in the Salzburg house where he later lived, you can read letters he wrote, including to his wife, Constanze. He is playful and practical and aware of money. He does not come across as a saint, and yet his musical gift is surely divine.

And then, there is *The Sound of Music.*

Austria may think this an appalling piece of kitsch but much of its tourism derives from it.

Because of COVID, there is just a shy cluster of six of us outside the Panorama kiosk in the center of the city. In usual summers, there would be a fleet of coaches, engines running. Now, there is one minibus and a stoical guide for the four-hour tour. And it is not even the minibus painted with scenes of Julie Andrews and children dancing through meadows that is parked opposite as a doleful advertisement.

The guide, a wry mother selling the von Trapp family idyll, says that in normal times, a busload of seventy passengers would leave twice a day for this tour. Now she is working four days a month and starting to sell off her possessions.

"Shall we sing?" she adds, brightly.

My fellow passengers follow her, waiting for the magic to begin. They include a honed blond Delta Air Lines stewardess— the only American crew flying. She brought a planeload of Germans home and then thought, why stay in Munich when you could do *The Sound of Music* tour in Salzburg?

She had done it once before with her family, and was now doing it again in memory of those good times.

On the seats next to me are a mother and daughter. Angelica is three years old and a bright, slithery charmer, in urban-print trousers and shoes. She sings "Do-Re-Mi," yawns because of her early start, and asks if we are going to meet Maria. Her mother was a graduate of the New York Jazz Academy, majoring in song and trombone.

At the end of the tour, she belts out a few notes of "Climb Every Mountain," but Angelica scolds her, putting her hand over her mother's mouth. The mother laughs with a shrug. "Now you know what happened to my musical career." Her own mother, a music teacher, did this tour, so they are reenacting it. "Granny couldn't come because of COVID," says Angelica, with an exaggeratedly sorrowful expression.

At the back of the bus are a German couple: an athletic, intelligent-looking woman and an amused male companion.

The guide and I start to discuss the huge gay audience for *The Sound of Music*, to the surprise of the German passengers. "Really? Really?"

"Oh yes," says the guide, starting to tap her foot. "Somewhere in my youth or childhood . . ." She breaks off and sighs. "The toilets are just round the corner for those who need them."

We are dealing with Hollywood and reality both in the film and the setting. Maria was indeed a governess sent from Nonnberg Abbey to look after the seven children of a naval captain. She became a nun after listening to Bach, so music was her route to spirituality.

On a point of history, the captain gave up his post because Austria lost its coast after the First World War. In 1938, Austria was annexed to Germany under Hitler and von Trapp was offered a high office, which he rejected. He, Maria, and the children decided to flee to the United States. They set off as if on a hike, then took trains through the Austrian Alps, crossing into Italy, Switzerland, France, Britain, where they boarded a ship to their final destination, America.

They did not in fact walk across the Untersberg mountain after escaping in a car from a musical concert. The guide chuckles over this solecism: "If they had gone over that mountain, it would have taken them straight to Bavaria and Munich. Hitler's Eagle's Nest in fact. Maybe that is why there was no sequel." Her other favorite solecisms pertain to the songs.

"'My Favorite Things'? Schnitzel with noodles? Nobody would eat that here. It should say schnitzel and potatoes. . . . As for the heartbreaker, Christopher Plummer's rendition of 'Edelweiss': 'Bless my homeland forever'—This is *not* our national song." And, she adds, "Christopher Plummer was dubbed—do you want a refund for the tour, now you know that?"

I say that I can just about bear it unless I discover that Julie Andrews is not singing either. "Oh yes, she sings, she sings," nods the guide.

We stop the bus to look down from a high vantage point at the cathedral city of Mondsee, located on a lake of the same name. There is another small group of tourists here, and one senior white man waves at Angelica's mother and points at his chest.

She peers at it and sees that it is a Black Lives Matter badge. "Thank you," she calls, giving a thumbs-up. She adds under her breath, "I thought he must have been another *Sound of Music* fan."

I am musing again on music and faith because I pick up at the Mondsee Cathedral—the film setting of *The Sound of Music* wedding—the book written by the real Maria von Trapp, called *Yesterday, Today and Forever.*

The cathedral was originally constructed as a Benedictine abbey in AD 748, and has since been restored with a baroque, pink-lined ceiling. It is gorgeously decorated, and I watch Angelica make her way round it hand in hand with her mother, her eyes the size of Communion plates. She stands in front of black-and-gold arches and a painting of angels, cherubs, and doves. Below it is a little statue of a crowned Black Madonna, holding Jesus, also crowned and in a Christening robe.

Angelica wants to dress up a bit herself. Next time I see her, she is coming out of a shop, her cool printed top and trousers replaced by a dirndl, the national costume of Austria. She does a twirl for me. I open Maria von Trapp's book once I am back on the bus. It is a slightly folksy juxtaposition of her own story with that of the Holy family fleeing from Herod.

Presumably to boost sales, the book has pictures of the von Trapp family between chapters. There is one particularly homely one of the children wearing sailor suits, lined up in order of their size. From the smallest on the left, it runs Martina, Johanna, Hedwig, Werner, Maria, Agathe, and Rupert.

The book takes a particular interest in the trade of Joseph. Salzburg is a city of wood carvers and Maria makes a plea to value carpenters and artisans. "Unfortunately, these things are dying out so fast that our children will only know about them through books." Her other homespun wisdom is that singing stops people from talking about their "problems"—a phenomenon that she regards as a modern disease. Perhaps she foresaw the age of therapy ahead.

It is the wisdom of the human heart that Maria writes about best; the suffering and the consolation.

The book ends with a sad letter that Maria wrote in April 1951. She describes the start of a concert tour on the West Coast, waving goodbye to her pregnant daughter Martina and her husband Jean. Martina had bought a carved wooden cradle from Salzburg, and next time Maria saw her, she expected to see a baby in it.

Once in California, Maria got a call. The baby had died in childbirth, and Martina's heart had stopped. Maria flew back. She lined her daughter's coffin with balsam twigs and flowers, and in an old Salzburg custom, said a prayer for the next person to die, reminding us that anybody could be taken at any time. She placed the baby in her mother's arms, and covered them both with Martina's bridal veil. She wrote: "And now with the words and the music of the Requiem, we understood again what is meant by the words 'Holy Mother Church.'"

I keep this chapter to myself, for the rest of the bus has launched into "High on a hill was a lonely goatherd." Rodgers and Hammerstein are our real guides to the von Trapp family.

The locations are a bit composite. Our bus went to Leopoldskron Castle, the setting for the lake scene where Maria and the children tumble out of the boat in front of the indignant captain.

But the place that I have come to see is Nonnberg Abbey. It is the soul of *The Sound of Music*. What makes Maria so interesting is that she was a nun. The abbey is the oldest nunnery in the German-speaking world, founded in AD 714. In real life, Maria married at the church here. The film has been and gone, the nuns remain.

The bus stops at the bottom of the hill for Nonnberg Abbey but nobody gets out. The guide points it out but says there is no time to visit it. The bus has a schedule to stick to and perhaps many who do this tour no longer find walking up steep hills so easy. But this is the cornerstone of my research so I will return.

Aho has asked me to dinner with his family. He wants me to meet his students of Aramaic at Salzburg University and to discuss his proposals for a school of Alexandria, a treasure house of Syrian literature. Aho is worried that we understand about saving things but not languages. Yet languages are identity. The Indian writer Arundhati Roy described Shakespeare as a traffic policeman in her country, constantly asserting the superiority of the English language. She highlights the loss of Urdu and Persian poetry.

There is an Urdu saying: "The head which today proudly flaunts a crown, will tomorrow, right here, in lamentation drown." Aho fears that Aramaic, the language of Jesus, will go the same way.

We meet him in Mozart Square—a medium-height, bespectacled, unassuming figure holding up an umbrella. What makes him distinctive is his smile, which radiates upward like sunrise. We order coffee and apple strudel, which he insists on paying for, although I fear for the salary of an academic in the field of Aramaic.

He shows us documents about his project. The front page, stamped confidential, announces the European Syriac Center, to protect and promote the Syro-Aramaic cultural heritage. It explains: Due to the war in the Middle East, most Suryoye (Syriac Christians, i.e., Arameans, Assyrians, Chaldeans) have been displaced from their homelands and had to flee. As a result, a unique cultural heritage is in danger of extinction.

I ponder this, and send an email later to Tony Blair and other Middle East romantics. Tony Blair's office asks for more detail, but I never hear back after that. The trail goes cold.

Aho is telling me about a trip he is making later in the month to Tur Abdin on the Turkish-Syrian border, to see the ruins of Dara (Anastasiuopolis). Tur Abdin is the heartland of Syriac Christianity, a place of refuge for the fleeing Syrian Christians.

I would love to go with him but am doing a final trip to the monasteries of Greece and dare not chance my luck with any more quarantine risks. I promise him that I will accompany him next time, before Christmas. I can sense Aho's ancestral longing and think of how faith folds into the lives of the dispossessed.

In the meantime, Aho would like us to meet his students and show us Saint Peter's Church and the famous catacombs and hermit caves. The church was founded in the seventh century, the catacombs carved into the rock with an Old Testament beauty.

Saint Peter's cemetery, lying between the church and the rock of the Mönchsberg, is a kind of Pearly Gates, with its garden of bright flowers, the elegant arches of the catacombs, and the stone and wooden hermit houses perched on the sheer rock. Aho turns around to check that I am following, and of course I think of *The Sound of Music* scene in which the family is hiding behind the graves, and the Nazi flashlight flashes above their faces. Saint Peter's Church feels quieter, more monastic than the grand Baroque of Salzburg or Mondsee.

We walk along the river, watching the raindrops on the water, toward Aho's center for Syriac studies. It is a building of faded splendor high on the riverbank, in need of restoration, for which he has raised money. Inside, we are ushered into a small, plain room and offered Syriac hot cinnamon cakes and Nescafé coffee.

A young, elegant-looking priest dressed in black enters the room. He is from Kerala, in India, which I discover is home to a community of Syrian Christians. In her essay on language, Arundhati Roy mentions that her mother is also Syriac Christian, from Kerala.

Other students enter, another from India, one from America, and another from Holland. We shift up on our little sofa to make room and I hope that it does not collapse. I ask the American student if there is a particular interpretation of the scriptures that comes from Syriac. He talks of the poetic theologian, the lyricism of the psalms. He is fluent in Aramaic.

Then the students invite us to join their service in a small chapel at the end of a corridor. We take a seat in a pew as they perform a repeated gesture of prostration before the altar. Then they gather in a circle and strike up an extended liturgical chant. A priest walks toward them, swinging incense from a censer. The chant begins again. It is recognizable as the Creed, while being something altogether other.

Afterward, amid broad smiles and friendly farewells, we leave the students to walk with Aho across the top of the hill that looks over the city. I ask if the service is a little like that of the Coptics. I cannot quite place it. He responds, a tiny bit reproachfully, that it is a lot more melodic; did I notice that?

It is getting autumnally dark and the rain is still spitting as we take the rocky hilltop path across to Nonnberg. Aho leads us through the trees, opening his heart. He is vexed by university politics and his inability to get Aramaic onto the agenda. I want him to succeed, but I know also that the Syriac monasteries do not feature much on the list of global priorities at the moment. And yet, in the monasteries, they are praying for the world and have plenty of wisdom to offer.

We reach Nonnberg Abbey and Aho's address, 1 Nonnberg, which compensates for many of his spiritual frustrations. The door to the house, which is somehow formed from the hillside, opens and his family are lined up slightly in the style of *The Sound of Music*.

Aho's wife, Penelope, is English, tall, rangy, intelligent. They met at Oxford and have led the life of academics ever since. Their three teenage children, two boys and a girl, Rachel, are a mix of savvy and observant. One of the sons is sporty, the other is arty. Rachel is spirited, challenging her father on the fact that she was sent to the kitchen during their last monastic trip while her brothers talked to the patriarch.

Aho is humorous, anxious, unworldly. Penelope is the balm of the family, moving effortlessly from teasing to tenderness. Aho says grace before the meal and the children bow their heads respectfully. And when Rachel talks about wanting to pursue a career as a dancer, she slips in that she would first like to spend some months staying in monasteries so that she can put her turbulent teenage years behind her and look ahead with a calm mind and still spirit. Aho looks across at her, beaming.

I have one more thing to do in Salzburg and that is to see, at last, Nonnberg Abbey. Aho says that there is a Communion service at 6:30 A.M. and he will ask the abbess if we can accompany him. The Benedictine nuns do not usually allow strangers into their services.

Next morning, at dawn, we climb the pathway and see Aho, freshly showered and smartly jacketed, waiting for us. "You came!" he says with his winning smile, which could charm the birds if not win grants from a vice chancellor.

We are back at the gates that the children shook in their attempt to speak to Maria in *The Sound of Music.* This time the gate is open, the bell is ringing, and the abbess greets us warmly at the church door.

The little church is lit up with sunrise, which casts patterns across the stone latticework on the ceiling. We follow the nuns up a small flight of stone stairs at the back of the church to find a secret chapel at the top.

Sitting in the choir stalls are the nuns, in wimples, black habits, and thick spectacles. One of them has a hacking cough. Another wheels in an elderly sister in a beret and woollen cardigan and parks the wheelchair at the end of the pew. The male priest is preparing the Communion with a young female altar server. Then the nuns begin their unaccompanied signing of the psalms, their voices youthfully pure, in contrast with their aging faces.

They line up with alacrity for Communion, for this is a closed community, protected from masks and sanitizers and panic. Then, with a bow from the priest, it is over, and we slip out through the side door, leaving the nuns for hours of further prayer. We see the altar girl whipping off her robes to reveal a polo shirt and jeans, and then hop on her bike and spin off to fetch croissants for her wife's (yes) breakfast.

I hug Aho goodbye outside the church. I hope that he gets his faculty of Aramaic. Below, Salzburg is stirring—the city of fortifications, spires, and Mozart—and up floats the early-morning noises of delivery vans and opening cafés.

I hum from the musical that we don't talk about. "My heart will be blessed with the sound of music and I'll sing once more. . . ."

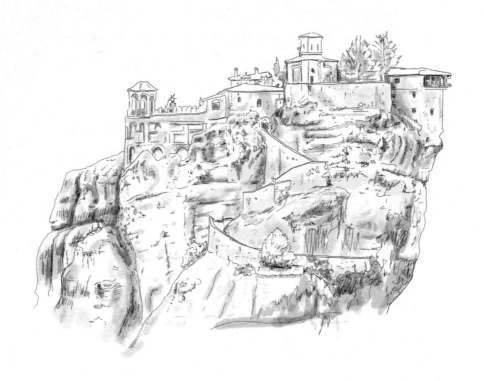

Chapter 10

HUMILITY AND SACRED QUIET

METEORA, GREECE

I am leaving my job as editor of the *Today* program. The addiction to news has become corrosive to me now that I have learned how to exist outside the news cycle. My nervous, distracted mind has experienced stillness. As W. B. Yeats wrote: "Bring the balloon of the mind/That bellies and drags in the wind/Into its narrow shed."

News is generally regarded as a form of enlightenment, but it is often just information wrapped in judgment, or worse, incitement. News demands drama and hyperbole. I remember when I was the editor of the *Sunday Telegraph* newspaper more than a decade ago, looking at a headline claiming local "fury" over a piece of planning permission. I remarked to the news editor that having read the quotes from residents it seemed more a case of mild irritation than fury. The news editor responded wryly: "*Irritation* isn't a headline word."

I find a little book about a celebrated monk who lived on Mount Athos and who warned against the intrusion of news.

Father Silouan was a Russian peasant born in 1866 who became a savant of the Eastern Orthodox Church. He settled on Mount Athos, the monastic peninsula in northern Greece, in order to contemplate the mystery of being.

According to Father Silouan, wisdom is based on humility, and he protested his ignorance if asked to pronounce on events. In other words, he was the antithesis of Twitter. He also had a view on print journalism:

> *The reading of newspapers darkens the mind and hinders pure prayer. . . . When the soul prays for the world, she knows better without newspapers how the whole earth is afflicted and what people's needs are. She can pity men without the help of papers.*

As a news journalist, I ponder the paradox. How can you pray on behalf of the world if you do not know what is going on in it? Father Silouan, however, was determined that he did not need to know. He understood that the human condition is capable of sorrow and joy, of virtue and sin. News reporting flows from this. The ubiquity of news media is a form of hubris, at odds with monasticism.

Enlightenment lies in self-renunciation. "I want only one thing," wrote Father Silouan, "to pray for all men as for myself." What this required was sacred quiet and the darkness of the night, which the Church fathers described as hyperluminous. Father Silouan's last words were: "I have not yet learned humility." He died shortly afterward, peacefully.

Humility does not come naturally to those of us in the chattering trades. Aggravated by social media, the journalistic impulse is exhibitionism and noise and entitlement. I admit to being guilty of all these when I realized that I was not permitted to visit Mount Athos. I read Patrick Leigh Fermor's account of it, and instead of admiring his surgeon's accuracy and poet's heart, I thought: "Well, it is all right for *you*."

I transferred my pity from myself to Rachel, the spirited daughter of my friend Aho. It was *outrageous* that she should be sent to the kitchens while her brother and father discussed faith with the elders. Is monasticism a patriarchal conspiracy?

Then I felt the still, small voice. It is not about *you*. It is not even particularly about monasteries, just this one. Some of the monks of Mount Athos left to form another monastic settlement, in some ways more spectacular. This is Meteora, a group of monasteries perched like eagles nests on the top of thrusting peninsulas in the mountains of Thessaly, in central Greece. There are both monks and nuns here in the monasteries in the air.

As I pack my familiar hand luggage of sample toiletries and look at the zig-zagging flight details—depart Luton, arrive Gatwick—I am also keeping a news eye on the quarantine lists. I cannot be too monastic about news at a time when countries are dropped onto a blacklist at a moment's notice. France is on the UK's banned list and the newspapers are speculating that Greece will be next. But there is still time. . . .

The pilgrims to Eastern Orthodox churches might have come from Russia, or Iraq, or Turkey. I come from Luton via easyJet. My fellow passengers to Thessaloníki, Greece's port city on a gulf of the Aegean, are vacationers, dispersing to the coastal resorts. They are pioneers of a sort, restless for sun and space.

The young jostle carelessly together (plague skeptics), while the older and more fearful jump into six-foot-distanced spaces. The plane lands in the late evening, in oily, blinking light and heat, and we while away some time in the car rental office at the edge of the airport.

"You drive," I say to my husband, forgetting my objections to the patriarchy. Then we are on the wide road to the city center, cars hooting humorously as we swing right mistakenly on a red light. Thessaloníki has a sweeping bay, and I see the Maersk containers lined up at the quay. This is a country of trade and conquests. It has been Byzantine and Ottoman, and has fought the Balkans and itself in civil wars.

Ancient Greece coexists with the Greece of vacationers. In Thessaloníki, the hotels are named Electra and Andromeda. And we are heading in the morning for Mount Olympus—seat of the Greek gods—and Meteora, home of monasticism. The story of Meteora is metaphorical as well as geological.

The hermits who wanted to climb toward heaven and later the Eastern Orthodox monks fleeing Ottoman Turks took refuge in this strange geological Jerusalem. Thirty million years ago, when there was a Lake of Thessaly, great boulders of sandstone and conglomerate mud deposits were formed from the trauma of the earth. Earthquakes and floods shook and fractured the landscape. Water pouring from gorges into the Aegean Sea split the sediment, creating a high-rise city of stone.

This is the historical evolutionary explanation: Ancient myths were added. This is the border between heaven and earth, just as it was the border between Greece and the Ottoman Empire. It was created out of the battle of Titans, when the gods of Olympus took on the gods of Thessaly, throwing rocks like javelins until they formed a citadel of stone pillars. Zeus, leading the Olympians, ordered his hundred-handed giants, the Hecatonchires, to uproot boulders and hurl them at the Titans. This explains the ugly/beautiful disorder of Meteora: misshapen boulders, some needle pointed, some bulky, some tumorous, hidden behind the restful hills of Thessaly.

I have recovered from my temper with Mount Athos, and we set off for Central Greece in our rental car, scribbled with undetected scratches and scrapes in the bright morning light.

Olympus is visible in the distance on the coastal road to Thessaly, and we take a sharp turn toward a mountain route for a closer look at Zeus's mountain. It has become humid and there are forecasts of storms. The sky is Aegean blue, eclipsed by gathering clouds as big as boulders. I keep an eye out for thunderbolts. We are sport for the gods.

It is a two-hour drive from Thessaloníki—or five hours if you choose to go through the Olympus Range. These roads are not arteries but veins, sometimes tangled or broken. The main road is a ribbon of developments strewn with garages, industrial yards, outlets, garden centers selling knockoff Greek statues. It has a Balkan feel to it, reminding me of the intertwined histories of Greece and Macedonia, or North Macedonia as the Greeks now call it.

The roads become steeper, the valleys turn to gorges and suddenly, as we reverse the shuddering car out of a dead end, Mount Olympus springs in front of us. I have not seen a mountain appear so spontaneously since Mount Fuji in Japan. Its white peak is behind feathery clouds but it is distinctively triangular. Its point is precise and neat, at 9,573 feet (2,918 meters), where Fuji flattens into a volcanic plateau at a grander 12,388 feet (3,776 meters). But both express a sacred quiet.

Around the corner, it is out of sight again. In search of a break, we find a road to a rural hamlet named, ambitiously, Petra. It is sleepy and peaceful in the midday heat. There is a small white roadside chapel with a little bell, some goats, and a tortoise crossing the road. There is no sign of any people, but a radio is audible from one of the back rooms beneath a red-tiled roof.

I get out to wander along the track, which leads back into the next swooping hillside. I pass some small horse chestnut trees, a fig tree, a chicken. The peak of Olympus is capriciously veiled behind a cloud.

My husband ("you drive!") would like to get on with the journey, for it is still two hours to Meteora. We take a look at a river, clear water over smooth pebbles, and I see my first person: a man asleep under a sycamore tree.

We reach Trikala in the afternoon, a little border town which was half Muslim, half Christian until the great exchange of religious populations in 1923. It was their partition and yet somehow because of its jumbled history, it is shrugged off as yet another conflict absorbed by Greece.

Trikala was built upon Trikka, mentioned in Homer's *Iliad* for its role in the Trojan War. History and myth are hard to separate in the Plain of Thessaly, domain of the river god Peneus, whose eponymous streams flow through it on their way to the

Aegean Sea. It is recorded as the birthplace of the healing god Asclepius, and here the monks medicine flourishes among pagan rocks.

We book into a spa hotel, except there is no spa because of COVID. The Ancient Greeks may have disported themselves naked in gymnasiums. These days we stick to social distancing and PPE.

Ancient Greece did not escape pandemics. There is a painting by the seventeenth-century Dutch painter Michiel Sweerts called *Plague in an Ancient City*, which depicts the plague of Athens as Judgment Day; figures draped and dying, illuminated and suffering. The plague in 429 BC killed the first citizen of Athens, Pericles, whom the British prime minister Boris Johnson keeps close to him in the form of a bust. I wonder if he thought of Pericles when he was taken into intensive care at St. Thomas' Hospital with COVID.

I walk from the hotel over a hilltop with panoramic views of fields and livestock on one side and the town of Trikala positioned on the other. It is a pilgrims' path, with a view far ahead of Meteora, a shape as distinctive as Olympus, a giant's mount, splintered into a second rock. I realize only the next day that this is not Meteora itself but simply the gateway to it.

A little distance from Meteora is a limestone rock from which flint and fire materials from the Neolithic period have been found. The sweep of history is laid out before me. I look up at the sun resting on the tips of the hilltops.

The angry Zeus clouds I saw earlier at Mount Olympus have changed here to soft Prussian blue and gray and, startlingly, peach. Above Meteora, the clouds are backlit. I think of the monks and nuns looking up from their mountaintop chapels to a celestial sky.

We leave for the monasteries the following day, as the sun rises behind us. Our guide, George, is from Trikala, and played as a child among the rock pillars, as if in a Greek myth. His brother, who kept sheep, used the hermit caves for shelter. George is wearing a blue polo shirt with sunglasses hanging from its collar, but despite his magazine appearance, he has a boyish quality. He picks up stones as if, like David, he might hurl them at the stone Goliaths.

We drive through the pretty bustling village at the foot of Meteora, which is more Lake District–style hiking shops than Lourdes souvenir iconography. The monasteries do attract pilgrims, but just as many hikers. They marvel at the beautiful scenery of plane trees and grassy knolls in the summer and endure the frozen snows and icy winds of winter.

The road loops behind the conglomerate mountain that I had seen from the hotel, and reveals, with a magician's flourish, the hidden world of Meteora. It is as if the Titans were turned to stone; elemental pillar statues, twisting and thrusting toward the sky.

The monks and the hermits made their way here in the eleventh century, and three centuries later, a monk named Athanasios from Mount Athos founded the first monastery. Another monk, Varlaam, built a second monastery on a tall rock opposite. They are compared to eagles nests but they are more like little castles; thick stone walls whose foundations are rock; ascension towers, from which baskets were winched down chains to bring the monks up. These are fortresses against the secular world and its values.

The monasteries of Meteora declined during the course of the seventeenth century and there are just six remaining: the Great Meteoron, Saint Varlaam, Holy Trinity, Saint Stephen, Saint Nicholas, and Rousanou.

Observant hikers may come across the ruins of others hidden in the hills and rock faces like a giant puzzle: the remains of the monasteries of the Highest in the Heavens, of the Calligraphers, of Saint John the Baptist, of the Holy Spirit, of Saint Peter's Chains.

We stop first at the foot of Meteora to look at the little eleventh- to nineteenth-century Byzantine Church of the Assumption of the Virgin. It seems modest from the outside, until George points out the embedded stones taken from the original Temple of Apollo. Here is the face of the sun, and a symbol of Genesis. The medieval Knights Templar, who journeyed to Jerusalem in search of the meaning of the universe, visited this church. The pagan is assimilated into the heart of the church. The font is built from the marble of Apollo's temple.

The history of Christianity is also marked here. The pulpit is in the center of the church, as it was in early Christian times. And the vivid murals depict Christian martyrdom at the hands of the Romans. The double-headed eagle is the symbol of empires, Roman and Eastern. The altar faces east, symbolizing sunrise and Jerusalem. The medieval world is framed in this little church, at the feet of floating monasteries.

The iconography of the fourteenth century is on display in all the monasteries of Meteora. It is there in scenes of torture, beheadings, and deathly figures hung from their feet. At the Great Meteoron and Varlaam, punishments become increasingly extravagant and grotesque. Heads of monks and saints, identified by rimmed gold, roll across the ground or are carried in bowls. Torsos drip blood. Men are flayed. Martyrs are eaten by lions.

There are two other prevailing images. One is the Day of Judgment. The scales are balanced; demons lead the damned off with ropes around their necks, while the saved ascend to heaven. Hell is heat, or ocean, where grotesque sea monsters await. The monks are praying for the salvation of humanity, but make full artistic use of a deterrent. Hell feels less theoretical in Meteora.

The other is the figure of Mary, who restores gentleness to the allegorical landscape. My favorite iconography in Meteora is the repeatedly drawn painting of Jesus at the coffin of Mary. He is holding her spirit, a newborn baby, symbolizing purity, and he is waiting to take her up to heaven with him. The Assumption of Mary is filial as well as Messianic.

We drive a little further up the winding mountain path, lined with trees of oak, plane, and birch. I look more closely at the gouged shapes in the rock and the smaller boulders, which, close up, resemble Henry Moore sculptures. They have been smoothed by the prehistoric rivers that tumbled into the Lake of Thessaly and on to the Aegean Sea.

And then I look again. Incredibly, a monastery has been built flat into a rock. Saint Gregory's is a hermitage with little wooden balconies and arched windows, created within sheer rock. Here is the little ladder that can be drawn up against invaders, there the window-sized door. On the balcony, there is movement of figures, men and women. These are the locals who go to assist the monk who lives there.

George says that the abbot of Saint Gregory's led the mon-astery of Holy Trinity further up in Meteora, but one day one of his monks decided to renounce his calling. This is a rare occur-rence and there are heavy penalties. The leader of the monastery must also leave, showing a responsibility that I cannot imagine being replicated by CEOs. So now the monk lives in his rock hermitage and takes confession among the locals. I ask George the name of the monk and he says: "We call him Old Man."

I shoot a skeptical look, but George is looking reverently up at the balcony. The monks are the repositories of wisdom, which is another word for truth. As Socrates told Aristotle: "Truly we have learned that if we are to have any pure knowledge at all, we must be freed from the body." The monks withdraw in order to pursue this knowledge. I wonder, is it the sacred quiet or the focus on liturgy over news that gives them their contemplative insights? The location, suspended between earth and sky, must be part of it.

Plato said: "Nothing ever is, everything is becoming. . . . All things are passing and nothing abides." The geological age of Meteora gives perspective to this summer of anxiety; and the contemplative calm of the monks an antidote to our present state of mind.

I run my hand along a gap in one of the rocks into which a hermit cave has been constructed with a wooden-barred gate to protect it. George demonstrates how you can start to build a hermitage, using vinegar, hammer, and nails. The vinegar softens the rock so that you can drive in a stake for use as a handle or a step.

The Monastery of the Transfiguration, or the Great Meteoron, is the first and largest of the monasteries, reached by 115 steps carved into the rock. It is the most famous visitor attraction in the area and usually you might expect to find coaches swaying up this hill. The pilgrims come from America, Russia, Australia, and the UK, but for now the tourists are from Greece, France, or Italy. All want selfies on the rock pillars. The ancient and the contemporary coexist. A sign advertises a pilgrims app. Meanwhile, the monks are glimpsed at the ticket office or in the chapels; they built the monasteries in the air to escape people but have reached an accommodation.

They earn enough from ticket sales to maintain the monasteries, and in return must give up sacred quiet for several hours a day. In the fourteenth century, Meteora monasteries were built with sanatoriums for the care of monks. There were fireplaces to keep them warm, and they were given natural remedies and hot beverages. Today, there are not enough monks to look after each other in sickness and old age and they seek help from villagers, who are very protective of them.

In the nineteenth century, the Greek government demanded that the relics from the monasteries—the liturgical books in gold leaf, the chalices and crosses and decorated robes—be taken to Athens for display. But when the officials arrived with their permits, they were driven back by the villagers. The people of Thessaly said they had protected the relics of Meteora for six hundred years of Ottoman rule and were not about to hand them over now.

The Great Meteoron is a collection of stone-and-brick buildings centered around a domed church. It was Athanasius who arrived here first, but the beautiful decorations of the church date to the sixteenth century. Images of the suffering of the saints depict men sliced and beheaded but radiating stillness. All things are passing, and nothing abides.

From the Great Meteoron, you look across to the next pillar supporting the monastery of Varlaam, and from there down to a lower boulder and the Rousanou nunnery.

Meteora, like Mount Athos, forbade the presence of women. But in the 1920s, a fire broke out in one of the monasteries, witnessed by women working in the vineyards below. They ran up to help and their bravery changed the hearts of the monks. There are now two nunneries in Meteora, Rousanou and Saint Stephen.

The heat is scorching as we wander from the Great Meteoron toward the rock pillar of Varlaam. The monasteries have different characters, and Varlaam feels lighter and more delicate. It is reached via a bridge and has small lawns, a vegetable garden, and a pleasant courtyard of trees, with a parachutist's view of the valley beneath. The church is movingly painted in the now-familiar scenes of persecution and heavenly judgment.

Sitting in one of the wooden stalls at the back of the church is a monk, in his black cassock and long beard. He is talking to a woman in the next stall, perhaps his sister. Their conversation is fond and punctuated by comfortable silence. Their gaze returns to the wall paintings. A young man approaches the monk, who warmly clasps his hand. While we visitors file anonymously through the church, obscured by our face masks, it is the monk who is the most animated and curious figure.

The third of the trinity of monasteries is the nunnery of Rousanou, dedicated to Saint Barbara, topically, the saint of contagious diseases. We approach the nunnery down a dappled woodland path. The Great Meteoron and Varlaam tower over us like independent city-states.

I like the meekness of Rousanou. There is a little garden with brightly colored plants laid out in a cross-shaped stone trough. The flagstone floor is spit-spot clean. A nun in a wooden ticket office averts her eyes as my husband pulls on a pair of one-euro paper trousers over his shorts. Modesty is another source of income for the monasteries.

Most of the relics of Saint Barbara lie in Venice, but some remain in this monastery. The nuns hope this might rub off on the visitors. A notice reads: "We hope and pray that the strenuous ascent to our monastery and to Holy Meteora will be spiritually uplifting and may become for you an opportunity to discover, feel, and draw near God."

Outside on the bridge, a couple pose for Meteora's thousandth selfie of the day. I repeat Plato's lesson: "Nothing ever is, everything is becoming." We try to capture time with our iPhones but the monks understand transience and flux. We cannot GPS our lives and fates. As Socrates said to his friends before drinking his fatal hemlock: "We go our separate ways—I to die and you to live. Which one is better God only knows."

It is as if Meteora deliberately defies photography. As soon as you steal a picture of a rock pillar, it has subtly changed its appearance, or its context. The light moves across the woods and hillsides and shadows change the colors of the boulders from rose to seal. The camera cannot see what the eye can see.

The superiority of the eye dictates monastic rules. No videos or photography. I wince as a young guy in shorts and T-shirt snaps away at the murals, while the painted saints look down in sorrowful humility.

In the evening, I go back to stand on the hill by the hotel and look across to Meteora. The shapes of the big and smaller rock are smudgier tonight, the sunset less fiery. It is as if Meteora has its finger to its lips.

I think of the words of the Victorian explorer Robert Curzon: "Nothing can be more strange and wonderful than this romantic region that is unlike anything I have ever seen before or since." Tomorrow I will return.

My dreams are empty that night, and in the morning I rise rested. I sit on the balcony for a while, watching the morning settle, and enjoy the sound of birdsong and the rustle of trees instead of the drill of breaking news.

Then we drive back toward Meteora. Again, I feel the thrill of the geology, passing that prehistoric limestone rock and seeing the lump of conglomerate that signals the entrance to the holy city.

Today we visit the loveliest monastery of all, Holy Trinity, which had been closed the day before. It looks unreachable from the road, except by a cable car, which crosses the steep ravine.

As we pull up in front of it, we see a monk climb into the cable car and whirr across to the peninsula. An abandoned scooter suggests the second part of his journey—the monks may be close to heaven but they are also pragmatic.

We find a path from the road, which leads us down to steps, hacked into the rock. The steps take us to the carved-out entrance to Holy Trinity. There is a strip of light up the center of the steps and everywhere light pours into the monastery. This is asceticism at its most aesthetic, monasticism packaged as a shoot for *Interiors* magazine. There is an emerald garden with limestone pots and containers placed in designer arrangements. Pink and yellow roses decorate the rock path into the building. The ascension tower is immaculate; even the winch hook looks as if it should be displayed in a design museum.

There are stone frieze decorations of mythical beasts, a red-tiled room with Roman-style arched brick work, so chic that it could be an art gallery. In the vestibule outside, there are a brightly restored pair of paintings of the Madonna and child, rimmed in gold, and of Jesus, his left hand raised and fingers pressed together in the sign of the Holy Trinity.

Another path leads you past watered and tended allotment gardens of tomatoes and salad leaves, to the top of the peninsula, for an eagle's view of Meteora. A white cross, planted in the stone, can be seen for miles. I am embarrassed by my enthusiasm for Holy Trinity. It seems to me a villa of my magazine dreams. Then I find a postcard of it in snow and imagine the bone-aching cold and loneliness of being a monk there. It would require the commitment of a hermit.

I leave Holy Trinity reluctantly but there is already quite a crowd heading for the end of the mountain road, to the Monastery of Saint Stephen. This has been a nunnery since 1961 and seems the best equipped as a visitor attraction. There is a wide easy-to-cross bridge rather than stairs. There are stalls selling bottled water. As you walk into the courtyard, you see rows of oak doors and iron bolts on two levels; this is home for the nuns but it also looks like a stage set. Saint Stephen is homely. The gardens are cared for. The chapel is a showcase, built in the columnar architecture of Mount Athos, and the sacristy a treasure of liturgy. The iconography of monks here is calligraphy and manuscripts.

As Aristotle knew: A fully human life is the activity of the mind.

Among the two busloads of European visitors arriving at the monastery, I spot a couple of monks apparently wandering down from their own monasteries. One, tall and handsome, is appreciatively watched by a cluster of female tourists, yet remains oblivious.

Another cheerful-looking monk picks up a small child and lifts him up to kiss the relics. The church contains the skull of Saint Charalambos, believed to cure illness, but it does not seem to alarm the child who holds out his arms. Monasticism may be imitation of the angels, but these monks can move within society and outside it. Their sights are beyond.

I have not learned humility yet but I have witnessed it in Meteora. The composure of the monks in company or alone reminds me of Archbishop Angaelos in Egypt. There is a serenity based on self-renunciation. The lack of self-assertion leads to an enlightened self. We demand self-realization and self-fulfillment. The monks demand—nothing.

Humility is not the same thing as surrender; it is acceptance. It is a word rarely used outside faith but as the difficult year of 2020 draws to an end, it is used by Boris Johnson. Johnson was a journalistic colleague of mine on the *Daily Telegraph* and he displays some journalistic habits in his role as prime minister. One is a limited attention span regarding a story. The COVID pandemic has dragged on too long. To begin with,

Johnson was quick to talk up cures and solutions but he has since come to terms with the fact that will and optimism are not enough. "We've got to be humble in the face of nature," he finally announces.

It is a monastic statement.

EPILOGUE

Meteora was the last trip I made and was the last one I would have been able to make. The UK is once again in lockdown and I am back in Norfolk. When I began my journey in search of stillness, nobody had heard of COVID-19. And yet the monastic message has chimed with the pandemic. Monks lived in the age of pestilence and they conceived self-isolation.

Confined at home, we have had to rely on inner resources, if not lockdown puppies. Deprived of society, we have confronted solitude and a different sense of time. The seasons have changed and the trees around my Cistercian wall are skeletal. All things are passing and nothing abides.

I have practiced a slightly more monastic rhythm of living. The turbulence of the American election took place under a harvest moon in Norfolk. While the media crowd on Twitter reported the election count by count, I took Joe Biden at his word and showed patience. I looked to the wall rather than at my phone. I searched for the interior silence.

I first heard this phrase on a windy November morning two years ago. My mother was suffering from an itchy arm wound and depression. I had heard that the nuns of Tyburn Convent in Hyde Park Place sold nun's balm, made from beeswax, lavender—and prayer. It was the only gift I could think of for flesh and spirit.

I hurried from the BBC offices at Portland Place, down Oxford Street, past Marble Arch, and on to the Bayswater Road. During that short walk, I looked at my phone several times: breaking news, terrorist attack in Melbourne; breaking news, forest fires in California—trolling Twitter, must phone parents. I was looking for a red-brick building with a small sign: Tyburn Convent, 8 Hyde Park Place, Shrine of the Martyrs.

There was no bell so I pulled at a door. Outside, heavy traffic and early Christmas shoppers paced. Inside, a chapel with a nun at prayer before the altar. She did not look up, and I hastily shut the door and fumbled for another entrance. A shutter opened and a smiling nun peeked out. I would like to see Mother Marilla, I said, trying not to sound like Julie Andrews.

Then I was seated in an office that resembled a local council waiting room, except for the rocking chair and a picture of the crucifixion on the wall. There was a plastic tablecloth on the cheap table, and on it, the smiling nun placed a tray for me with a glass of tap water and a plate of three rich tea biscuits.

Mother Marilla arrived. She is of Singaporean and Hong Kong heritage and has a marked Australian accent and a friendly face. Her ancestors were Buddhists; she is Catholic. She is accompanied by a smaller nun, whom she calls the "organizer."

Mother Marilla became a nun at twenty-four. She was reluctant to give up her old life: "I wanted to marry and to have children, I love life, I didn't want to be a nun." But then, she says, a great peace had entered her heart and she had given herself up to it. Whenever she leaves the convent she yearns to return to its peace.

Mother Marilla tells me she fears that those of us in the busy world might mistake the structured thought of monasteries for boredom. The first thing that is taught in monasteries is not to waste time. That is why, traditionally, monks and nuns have grown food, run farms, gardened, read books, tended the sick, while also praying throughout the day. Oh yes, and they also invented Dom Perignon and Benedictine liqueur.

The Tyburn nuns busy themselves making and packaging nun's balm. And then, from the evening to the morning, there is always monastic silence. Mother Marilla says that this is when the nuns find the deepest peace. "If you are not talking, you start to listen." This is the interior silence.

Mother Marilla believes that the distinguishing torment of modern life is noise. Everybody talking, nobody listening. "The mind is so distracted by noise."

At one point, during our conversation about her early life in Australia, she turns to her fellow nun and asks if she wants to do something else. I wonder if this is a coded message but it turns out to be something simpler and more unusual. Mother Marilla has sensed, despite no outward sign at all, that the nun is perturbed. It is the interior silence that bestows the gift of what we would call emotional intelligence and what Mother Marilla would call, simply, listening.

"Silent" is an anagram of "listen." It is how I shall try to live my life, as the monks have taught me. Attentive to the interior silence.

SELECTED BIBLIOGRAPHY

Agoritsas, Dimitrios K. 2013. *Meteora: The Holy Monasteries as a place of pilgrimage*. Kalampaka, Greece: Holy Monastery of Varlaam.

Alfeyev, Hilarion. 2003. *The Mystery of Faith*. London: Darton Longman & Todd.

Beckett, Wendy. 2013. *Spiritual Letters*. London: Bloomsbury Publishing.

Cassian, John. 1985. *Conferences*. New York: Paulist Press.

Covell, Stephen G. 2005. *Japanese Temple Buddhism*. Honolulu: University of Hawaii Press.

Culadasa (John Yates) and Matthew Immergut with Jeremy Graves. 2017. *The Mind Illuminated*. New York: Simon & Schuster.

De Gregorio, Scott, ed. 2006. *Innovation and Tradition in the writings of The Venerable Bede*. Morgantown: West Virginia University Press.

Fermor, Patrick Leigh. 2007. *A Time to Keep Silence*. New York: NYRB Classics.

Greene, J. Patrick. 1992. *Medieval Monasteries*. Leicester, UK: Leicester University Press.

Holland, Tom. 2019. *Dominion*. New York: Little, Brown.

Ignatius of Loyola. 1997. *Saint Ignatius of Loyola: Personal Writings*. Translated by Joseph Munitiz and Philip Endean. New York: Penguin Classics.

Jamison, Christopher. 2006. *Finding Sanctuary: Monastic Steps for Everyday Life*. Collegeville, MN: Liturgical Press.

Kavanaugh, Kieran, and Otilio Rodriguez. 2010. *The Collected Works of St. John of the Cross*. Washington, DC: ICS Publications.

Lainati, Chiara Augusta. 1994. *Saint Clare of Assisi*. Translated by Jean Frances. Assisi, Italy: Edizioni Porziuncola.

Laird, Martin. 2006. *Into the Silent Land: The Practice of Contemplation*. New York: Oxford University Press.

The Lives of the Desert Fathers. 1981. Translated by Norman Russell. Piffard, NY: Cistercian Publications.

Mantel, Hilary. 2020. *The Mirror and the Light*. New York: Henry Holt & Company.

Marshall, Peter. 2009. *The Reformation: A Very Short Introduction*. New York: Oxford University Press.

Mosebach, Martin. 2019. *The 21: A Journey into the Land of Coptic Martyrs*. New York: Plough Publishing House.

Nicoloff, Philip L. 2007. *Sacred Kōyasan,* New York: State University of New York Press.

Provatakis, Theocharis M. 1991. *Meteora: History of the Monasteries and Monasticism*. Toubis Editions.

The Qur'an. 2008. Translated by M. A. S. Abdel Haleem. Oxford, UK: Oxford University Press.

Radcliffe, Timothy. 2020. *Alive in God: A Christian Imagination*. New York: Bloomsbury Continuum.

Ratisbonne, Theodore. 1991. *St. Bernard of Clairvaux*. Charlotte, NC: Tan Books.

Rinpoche, Sogyal. 2020. *The Tibetan Book of Living and Dying*. San Francisco: HarperOne.

Rodríguez, Josep Liz. 2019. *Montserrat, the Sacred Mountain*. Translated by Mark Waudby. New York: Triangle Books.

Roswell, Roger. 2012. *The Medieval Monastery*. London: Shire Publications.

Ryan, John. 1972. *Irish Monasticism: Origins and Early Development*. Dublin: Four Courts Press

Stanley, Thomas. 2010. *Pythagoras*. Jersusalem: Ibis.

Thom, Catherine. 2008. *Early Irish Monasticism*. New York: T&T Clark.

Thubten, Gelong. 2019. *A Monk's Guide to Happiness*. New York: St. Martin's Publishing Group.

Trapp, Maria A. 1952. *Yesterday, Today and Forever: The Religious Life of a Remarkable Family*. Philadelphia: Lippincott.

Trapp, Maria A. 2001. *The Story of the Trapp Family Singers*. New York: Doubleday.

Varden, Erik. 2018. *The Shattering of Loneliness: On Christian Remembrance*. London: Bloomsbury Continuum.

Ward, Benedicta. 2003. *The Desert Fathers, Sayings of the Early Christian Monks*. London: Penguin Books.

Welch, John W. 1996. *The Carmelite Way: An Ancient Path for Today's Pilgrim*. Paulist Press.

ACKNOWLEDGMENTS

I wish to thank the supercharged sisterhood at Short Books: Aurea Carpenter, Kate Hubbard, Evie Dunne, and Katherine Stroud for their professionalism and decency and especially to Rebecca Nicolson for commissioning this book.

Thank you to all those whom I met on my travels and particularly the monks and nuns who endured the shallow questions of someone peeping into their lives.

Thank you to my beloved husband, Kim; and children, Henry, Rafe, and Tilly.